SIMPLE

TYPE 2 DIABETES COOKBOOK

FOR BEGINNERS

Simple steps to Managing Prediabetes & Type 2 Diabetes with

2000+ Delicious Days of Low-Carb & Low-Sugar Recipes. Includes

30-Day Meal Plan for Building Healthy Habits

PAULA J. EVANS

TABLE OF CONTENTS

CHAPTER EIGHT: VEGETABLE 168

CHAPTER NINE: SNACK 181

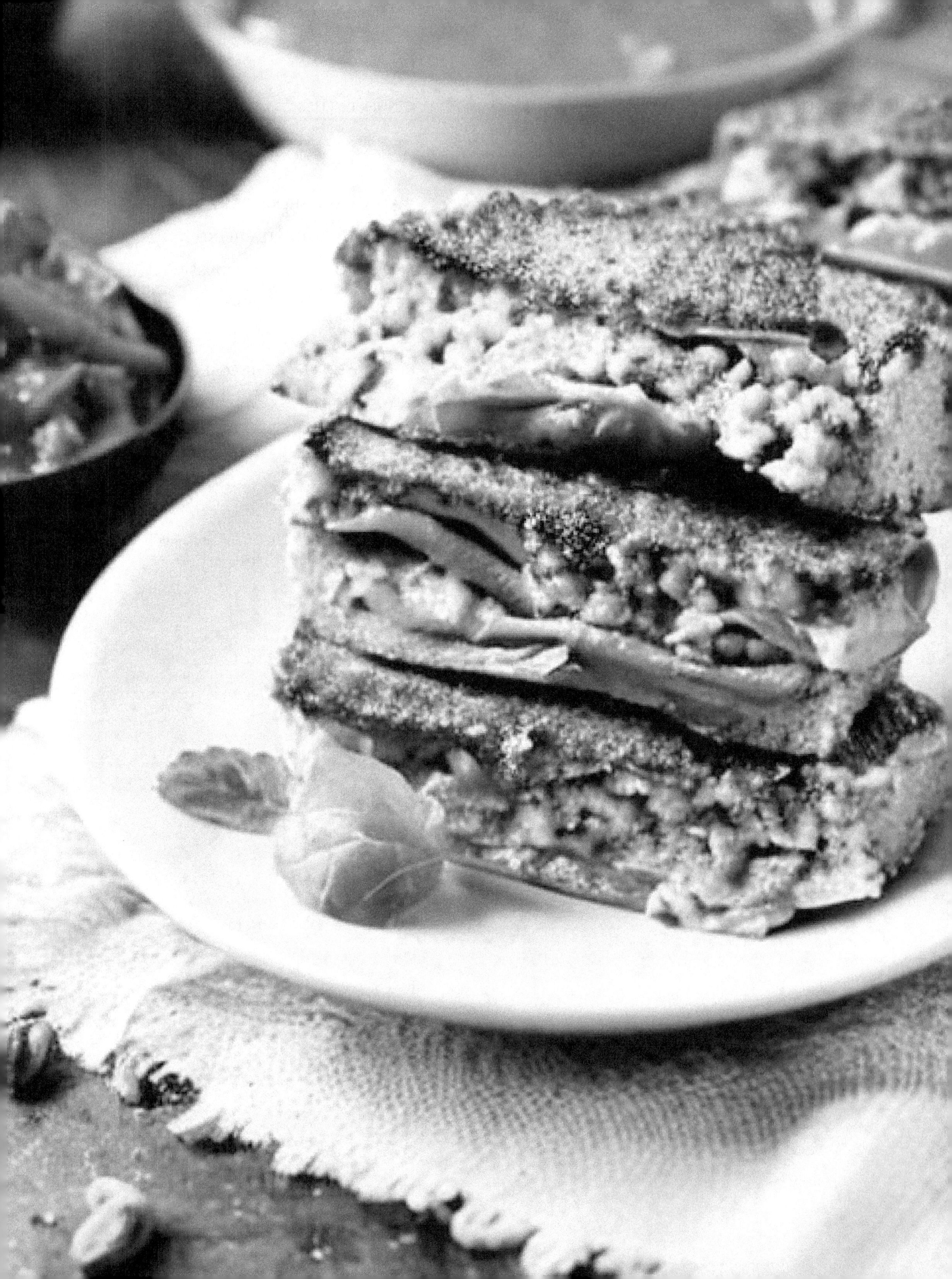

Diabetes is a highly dangerous condition that impacts how your body processes food into energy. Most of the food you consume is utilized to make glucose, which is subsequently released into your circulation. Your pancreas is in charge of managing your blood sugar. When blood sugar rises, it sends a signal to create insulin. Insulin functions like a key that permits blood sugar to enter cells and be utilized as energy. Having diabetes might imply that you do not create enough insulin, or the amount of insulin your body makes is not being utilized effectively. When your body is not manufacturing enough insulin or when your cells cease reacting to insulin, a significant quantity of blood sugar stays in your bloodstream.

You must be aware of all the symptoms and early warning indications that appear with this health issue if you have diabetes, or if you are at risk for getting diabetes. Living a healthy lifestyle may help prevent diabetes in the long term, particularly if it runs in your family. Simple lifestyle adjustments may also help you prevent or reverse prediabetes. Changes such as consuming better food, exercising more regularly, and Dropping weight if you're overweight may make all the difference. Some programs may also aid you with establishing lasting healthful changes in your life, such as

the CDC-led National Diabetes Prevention Program. Diabetes does not have a cure. If you don't take care of yourself, you may have more significant health concerns such as heart disease, eyesight loss, or renal illness. You must take your medicine and attend all healthcare appointments to reduce the effect of diabetes on your life. You may also get diabetic self-management instruction and support, which may aid you take care of yourself better.

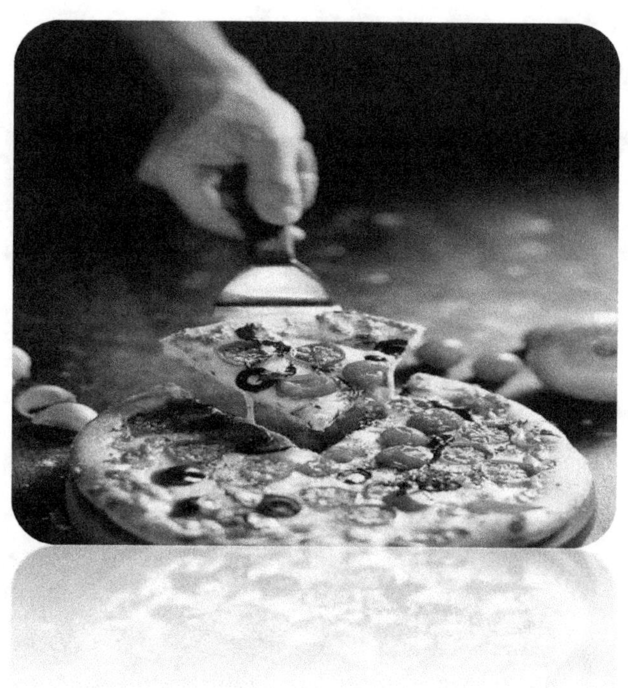

Knowing that you, your kid, or someone you love has diabetes may be harsh and upsetting. However, you should realize that there are numerous things you can do that can help manage the illness. Even with diabetes, you may live a regular life and go about your everyday activities - as long as you know to be fully prepared for an insulin emergency. Having diabetes does not mean that you can't still accomplish your greatest life goals. There are numerous Olympic athletes, football players, actors, politicians, and those that have diabetes - yet it never stopped them from achieving their aims. They live a healthy lifestyle that helps them control diabetes and if you do the same, you can thrive. Bringing physical activity into your regular lifestyle and eating better is the greatest strategy to control this illness.

This is why we created this book: to assist you manage your diabetes and prosper in life.

You and Diabetes

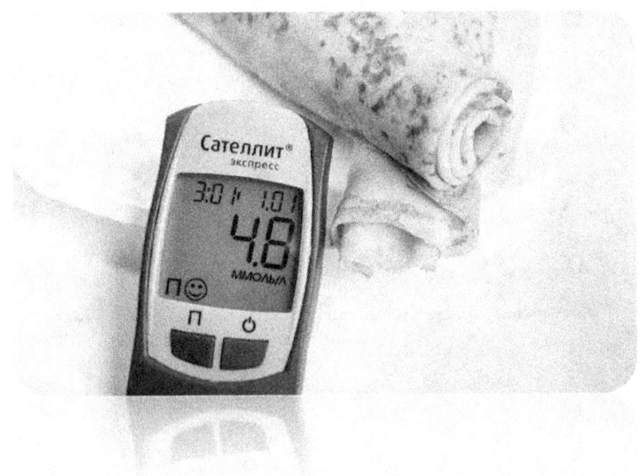

It may be quite upsetting to find that you or a family member has diabetes. Not only might you get anxious, but your whole family might, too. You may have so many questions. How much are medical bills? What can happen while you're not at home? Where can you receive adequate medical care? You can find yourself suddenly feeling like you're carrying the weight of the whole planet on your shoulders. Be cautious not to overthink; don't imagine for a second that your life is over or that you will just be recalled as "sickly." This is not the case. You are not alone. Many techniques exist that may help you and your family manage diabetes and help you live a happy, long, and healthy life.

Help Suggested

When you or a someone you love is diagnosed with diabetes, you may be at a lost unsure where to begin. Living with a medical condition may be incredibly tough, but you should realize that many individuals can support you. Consult a doctor about what you can do to keep safe and healthy. Inquire about different diets and lifestyle modifications you may need to undertake. Make touch with any friends or family members who have been impacted by this sickness. Talk to individuals on the internet who are going through similar experiences. You are now officially a part of an international community, and seeking out for assistance and support is the first step toward your new, healthy life.

Increase your Physical Activity

Physical exercise is vital for diabetes control. You must aim to be as active as possible. You don't have to spend two hours every day at the gym; just participating in 30 minutes or more of moderate physical exercise for the majority of the week may make a great impact. Increased physical activity may help you substantially decrease your blood glucose, cholesterol, and blood sugar levels.

Exercise may also boost your mood, self-esteem, and sleep quality while lowering stress and anxiety. Increasing your physical activity may also help strengthen your muscles and bones. If your doctor suggests that you lose weight, strive for at least an hour of physical activities most days of the week. It may appear to be a lot at first, but you may split it throughout the course of the day in short pieces of 10-15 minutes.

Improving your resistance is also highly encouraged, particularly if you have diabetes. You may speak with an exercise physiologist who can assist construct a safe resistance exercise regimen for you. Make it a habit to engage in resistance training at least twice a week. Push-ups, squats, and lunges are examples of resistance exercises. If you wish to workout at home, you can also use dumbbells and resistance bands. Lifting, lugging, or excavating doing domestic activities might also enhance your resistance. If you have the time and money, you may also join a gym and perform weightlifting and other resistance workouts.

To enhance your physical activity, you must also minimize the quantity of time you spend sitting at work or home. You may integrate physical activity into the day by adopting minor adjustments such as taking the stairs instead of the elevator or parking farther away from work so you may walk there. You may also take your dog, children, or grandkids for a stroll in the park. You can do your cleaning while watching television. You can also get off the bus one stop sooner and walk the rest of the way. There are countless strategies to include physical exercise into your everyday routine. You don't require to join a gym; merely modifying your activity will enough.

Diabetes and Support Programs

Diabetes is not something you can switch off when it is convenient for you. It must be monitored 24 hours a day, seven days a week. If your youngster has diabetes, check at diabetic support programs that may aid your kid in controlling their diabetes throughout the day. Since you cannot always be with them while they are in school or participating in school activities like as school excursions, summer camps, and leisure activities, students must learn how to respond in case of an emergency.

Under federal law, kids with diabetes have the same right as any other kid to get the attention they need to be safe and engage in school activities. With this, you should guarantee that your child's school delivers workers that have been educated in blood sugar (glucose) monitoring and insulin and glucagon administration, as well as professionals that have been trained to providing diabetic care on school excursions, during extracurricular activities, and at all school-sponsored events. In addition, your youngster must be able to handle their diabetes independently at any time and any place.

As a consequence, the schools where your children go should be able to aid in controlling your child's diabetes. You should not be compelled to go to the school in order to care for your child's diabetes. Along with that, your youngster should not be sent to a separate school to obtain required diabetes care, nor should they be banned from participating in school-sponsored activities.

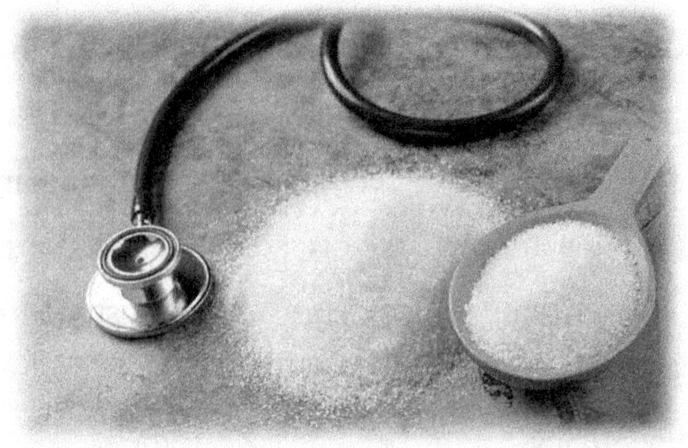

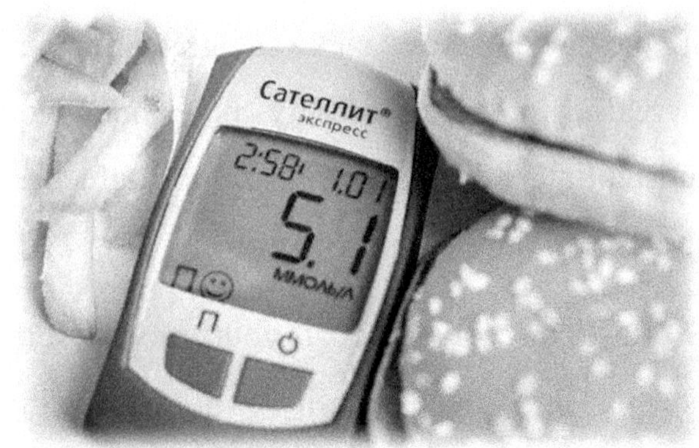

Diabetes is divided into three types: type 1, type 2, and gestational diabetes, which may develop in a woman during pregnancy. Aside from the three primary categories, some persons may additionally develop prediabetes, a disease in which someone's blood sugar levels are larger than usual but not high enough to be diagnosed with type 2 diabetes.

TYPE 1 DIABETES

Experts believe that type 1 diabetes begins when the body mistakenly assaults itself, limiting the body from creating the insulin that is essential help reduce blood sugar levels. Type 1 diabetes affects around 5-10% of persons with diabetes. Increased thirst, increased urination, excessive hunger, weariness, and blurred.

Here are some of the frequent symptoms of untreated type 1 diabetes. Type 1 diabetes symptoms may emerge gradually or quite rapidly. To live with type 1 diabetes, a person must take insulin on a regular basis. It is uncertain how to avoid type 1 diabetes, and the risk factors are not as evident as they are for type 2 diabetes and prediabetes. However, some recognized risk factors for type 1 diabetes are as follows:

- ❖ If you have a family member with type 1 diabetes
- ❖ Being at the age when type 1 diabetes most usually arises (anyone may acquire type 1 diabetes regardless of age, although it is most prevalent in adolescents, teens, or young adults)

TYPE 2 DIABETES

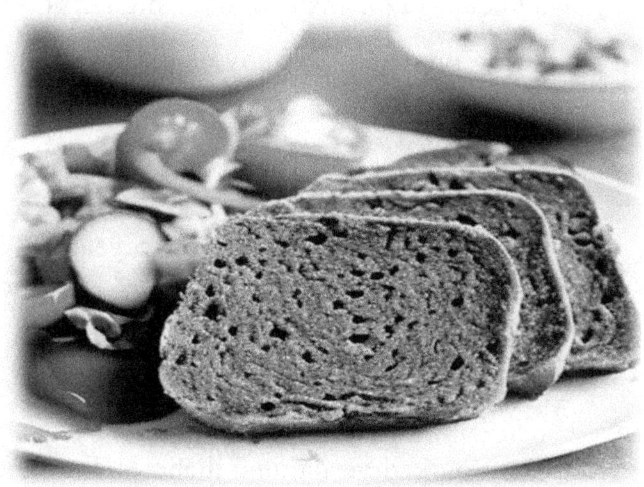

Type 2 diabetes is not the same as type 1. When you have type 2 diabetes, your body does not utilize the insulin it generates effectively, meaning that it cannot sustain regular blood sugar levels. Type 2 diabetes impacts roughly 90-95% of persons who have diabetes. It normally takes many years to develop and is most frequent in adults, however it is getting more seen in adolescents, teens, and young people today. Type 2 diabetes may not display signs at first, which is why it is crucial should get your blood sugar checked if you are at risk. It may be avoided or postponed by implementing healthy lifestyle adjustments such as increasing physical activities and eating healthy meals. The following are known type 2 diabetes risk factors:

- ❖ Presence of prediabetes
- ❖ Being overweight
- ❖ Age 45 years old or older
- ❖ Someone with type 2 diabetes is in your family
- ❖ Not being physically active
- ❖ You had gestational diabetes or given birth to a baby weighing
- ❖ over 9 pounds
- ❖ Being diagnosed with non-alcoholic fatty liver disease

GESTATIONAL DIABETES

Gestational Diabetes may occur in pregnant women even if the woman having no history of diabetes or prediabetes. The infant may be more vulnerable susceptible acquiring the illness if the mother has gestational diabetes. It normally resolves itself after your baby is delivered, although it does raise your odds of acquiring type 2 diabetes later in life. Your baby may also develop health issues such as obesity as a kid or teenager, and they are more prone to acquire type 2 diabetes later in life. You may be at risk of developing gestational diabetes while pregnant if you have any of the following characteristics:

- ❖ Gestational diabetes was present in a prior pregnancy
- ❖ Had a baby weighing more than 9 pounds
- ❖ Are overweight
- ❖ Are above the age of 25
- ❖ Have a family member with type 2 diabetes.
- ❖ Have been diagnosed with polycystic ovarian syndrome (PCOS)
- ❖ Are of African American, Hispanic/Latino American, American Indian, Alaska Native, Native Hawaiian, or Pacific Islander descent

If you lose weight, eat better, and exercise frequently before becoming pregnancy, you may be able to prevent gestational diabetes. While gestational diabetes is not permanent, the mother and baby may be at a heightened risk of acquiring type 2 diabetes later in life.

PRE-DIABETES

Prediabetes is fairly frequent, especially in the United States. It affects around 88millionadults, or more than one-third of all adults. Most people are unaware that they have prediabetes.

Prediabetes is described as having blood sugar levels that are more than normal but not quite high enough to be categorized as type 2 diabetes. If you have prediabetes, you are more likely to acquire type 2 diabetes. The dangers of other health conditions like heart disease and stroke are also elevated. The good news is that prediabetes may typically be reversed if you make the essential lifestyle adjustments. You may be at a high risk of acquiring prediabetes if any of the following applies:

- ❖ You are overweight
- ❖ You are above the age of 45 years
- ❖ A member in your family has type 2 diabetes
- ❖ You are not physically active
- ❖ You had gestational diabetes during a pregnancy
- ❖ You had a baby weighing more than 9 pounds
- ❖ You are of African American, Hispanic/Latino American, American Indian, Alaska Native, Asian American, or Pacific

Islander descent.

CHOOSING YOUR DIET

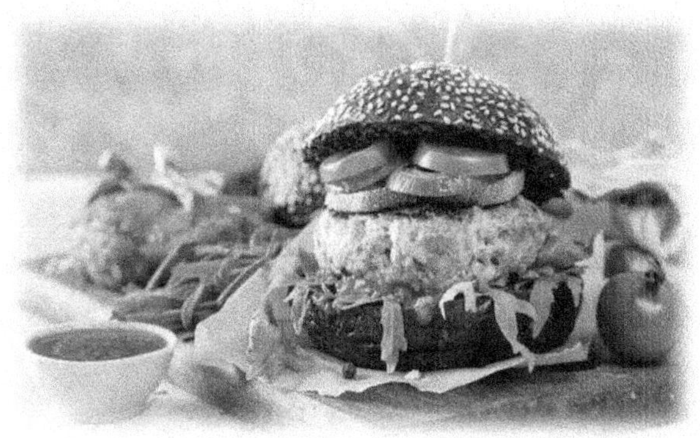

Your doctor may encourage you to contact a trained nutritionist if you are diagnosed with diabetes or prediabetes. Most nutritionists will suggest that you embark on a diabetic diet, and they may also help you build a healthy eating plan that is ideal for you and your requirements. A tailored eating strategy may help you regulate your blood sugar levels, maintain your weight, and minimize risk factors for heart disease.

A diabetic diet consists of three regular meals a day. This enables you to make better use of the insulin your body generates or that you acquire via medicine. A trained dietician may establish dietary programs that are customized for your individual health goals, interests, and lifestyle. They can give your ideas on how to modify your eating habits, such as how to regulate your servings to ensure they are suitable for your weight and activity level.

Eating too many calories and fat might contribute to a spike in blood sugar. If this is not managed, you may develop major health conditions such as diabetes retinopathy, nephropathy, macro vascular disorders, and more.

Additional long-term problems such as nerve, renal, and heart damage may also occur. It's vital that you be conscious of what you are putting into your body. Make smart meal choices and keep track of your eating habits to keep your blood sugar levels at a healthy range.

PRIMARY GUIDELINES FOR A DIABETIC DIET

A healthy eating plan might be highly useful if you have diabetes. If you chose to follow one, consider the following:

- Throughout the day, eat at regular intervals.
- Include veggies in every meal. Do your utmost to fill half of your plate with veggies that are not starchy.
- Make the size of your meals and snacks smaller.
- Include a little dose of carbs that are rich in fiber with every meal. Examples include brown rice, potatoes, whole grain bread, and whole grain pasta.

- Choose low-fat dairy products. Try to seek for some that do not contain a lot of additional sugar.
- Consider other lean meats and alternatives such as skinless chicken and turkey, fish, eggs, and tofu.
- Decrease the quantity of saturated fats in your meals by decreasing stuff like butter, processed meats, and fried meals. You can replace them with healthy ones such as olive, canola, or sunflower oil, avocados, and unprocessed lean meats.
- Be careful to incorporate fatty fish in your diet such as salmon, sardines, and tuna at least two to three times every week.
- Only consume sweets on rare occasions.
- Avoid candy and sugary beverages.
- Limit your consumption of salt and any items that are too salty.
- Consider using various herbs and spices to guarantee your cuisine does not taste dull.
- Limit alcohol consumption.

RECOMMENDED FOODS

If you have diabetes, you must learn to be more careful of the meals you eat. It may seem challenging at first; nevertheless, you'll learn that living a healthful lifestyle is definitely more rewarding in the long term. Going on a diabetic diet does not mean you have to consume dull and tasteless food. There are numerous tasty dishes that are perfect for diabetes. We've compiled a list of suggested items to include in your diet plan, as well as certain meals to avoid, in this chapter.

"Good" Carbohydrates

Carbohydrates are separated into two types. Simple carbs (sugar) and complex carbs (starch). Simple carbs can either be natural sugar that is generally present in fruits and milk or processed sugar that is present in soda and sweets. Complex carbohydrates, on the other hand, allude to entire grains, legumes, and vegetables. Sugar and starch are the two elements that are broken down into glucose.

If you have diabetes, it is crucial that you focus on healthy carbs such as:

- Fruits
- Vegetables
- Whole grain cereals
- Legumes like beans and peas
- Low-fat dairy products like milk and cheese

Fibrous Foods

Eating food that is rich in fiber may lessen the risk of several health diseases such as heart disease, constipation, and of course, diabetes.

Fiber is used to manage blood sugar levels by slowing down digestion. Fiber-rich foods include:

- Vegetables
- Fruits
- Nuts
- Legumes (such as beans and peas)
- Whole grains

Oily Fish

A diet that contains fatty fish has been connected with a lower risk of cardiac illness. Certain fish supply omega-3 fatty acids and include creatures like as tuna, sardines, salmon, and mackerel. If you have diabetes, you should take oily fish at least twice a week. It is also good for pregnant or nursing moms to do so since it enhances the baby's immune system.

"Good" Fats

Fats are typically avoided in many diets, yet there are specific fats that are helpful when taken rarely, especially for persons with diabetes.

Monounsaturated and polyunsaturated fats are plentiful in foods like as avocados, nuts, canola, olive, and peanut oils. These kinds of fats help decrease cholesterol. However, it is still crucial to note that fatty meals are rich in calories and should be taken in moderation.

FOODS TO AVOID

When you have diabetes, your chances of having additional health diseases such as heart disease or stroke are elevated. The following are several food categories that you should avoid if you wish to lower the danger of additional diseases and consequences connected with type 2 diabetes:

- **Saturated Fats:** Products that are heavy in fat and proteins such as butter, bacon, sausages, hot dogs etc. should be avoided. You should also minimize your usage of coconut and palm oil.
- **Sodium:** Your doctor would most likely advise you to have less than 2,300 mg every day if you have high blood pressure.
- **Trans Fat:** Trans-fat that is present in processed foods, baked products, and margarine should be avoided.
- **Cholesterol:** Dairy products and proteins that are rich in fat, like well as organ meats like egg yolks and liver are rich in cholesterol. In order to maintain a healthy lifestyle, you must restrict your daily cholesterol consumption to no more than 200 mg. Our food choices have a major

influence on our wellness. As we experience life, we must be aware of what is healthy and what is not. By becoming more mindful, we can lower the likelihood of having diseases or health concerns later on in life.

Processed Carbohydrates

Carbohydrates that have been treated have been devoid of their nutritious bran and fiber, as well as vitamins and minerals. White flour, sugar, and white rice are examples of processed "enriched" carbs.

Consuming too much processed carbohydrates might increase blood sugar and insulin rises. As you approach older, you are substantially more prone to get type 2 diabetes. White bread, sweet baked treats, and white pasta should also be reduced since they might cause a rise in blood sugar if ingested in excess. Be aware of things that are advertised as being "enriched" for the same purpose.

Sugary Drinks

A 2010 research published in Diabetes Care found that consuming more than one sugary drink per day has been demonstrated to raise the risk of type 2 diabetes by 26%1 Even if you don't believe you're at risk of having diabetes, it is vital that you limit your consumption of sugary beverages. To remain hydrated, drink additional water. In addition, you should avoid adding sugar and cream to your coffee or tea.

Saturated and Trans-Fat

Although not all fats are unhealthy for you, saturated and trans fats should be avoided. These facts are toxic and may elevate cholesterol levels in the blood. Saturated fats are often present in fatty foods, cheese, butter, and milk, but trans fats are prevalent both in packaged meals and fried dishes. Because having high cholesterol is a risk factor for type 2 diabetes, these fats should be avoided.

Red and Processed Meat

It's been proved that excessive intake of red and processed meat is related with type 2 diabetes. For instance, bacon, hot dogs, sausages, and other processed meats are examples of processed foods to avoid. These are particularly dangerous for you since they contain a lot of salt and nitrites.

CREATING A DIABETIC DIET PLAN

A diabetic food plan might aid you in maintaining normal blood sugar levels. You might employ a professional dietician to build a tailored meal strategy for you depending on your tastes and lifestyle. There are countless sorts of meal programs offered.

This meal planning strategy was created by the American Diabetes Association. This strategy encourages individuals to eat more veggies by arranging your dish in the following ways:

- ❖ Half of your plate should be made up of non-starchy veggies.
  Tomatoes, carrots, and other vegetables come under this group.
- ❖ Protein should account for about one-quarter of your meal. This might be an oily fish, lean meat, or skinless beef.
- ❖ Whole grains should make up roughly one-quarter of your dish.
  These might include brown rice or a starchy vegetable.
- ❖ Remember, eating in moderation is crucial when it comes to healthy fats.
- ❖ Include some fruit or dairy items, as well as a glass of water, tea, or coffee.

Counting Carbohydrates

Carbohydrates are thought to have the largest influence on your blood sugar level since they are the dietary category that is turned down into glucose. It is crucial that you understand how to measure your carbs in order to adequately regulate your blood sugar. This might also help you alter your insulin dosage appropriately. You may learn to calculate meal servings and read food labels with the aid of a skilled nutritionist. You should also consider learning about serving size and carbohydrate content.

Choose Your Foods

A professional nutritionist may propose particular meals that might benefit you in meal and snack planning. With this system, you may pick items from a range of categories such as fats, carbs, and proteins. Your "choice" is a single serving within a category. It must have approximately the same quantity of carbs, protein, fat, and calories as any other food in the same category. It must also have the same influence on your blood glucose levels.

Glycemic Index

The glycemic index is commonly used by a lot of people with diabetes for choosing food, particularly carbohydrates. This method ranks the effect of foods that contain carbohydrates on your blood glucose levels. It is best to consult a professional dietitian before trying this method to determine if it is right for you.

IMPORTANCE OF DIABETIC DIET

The absolute best way to control your blood glucose levels is by sticking to your healthy eating plan. By doing so, you can reduce your risk of developing further complications that diabetes may bring. You may also tailor your meal plan according to your needs, so it would be really helpful if you're planning to lose weight or if you have a specific health goal you want to achieve.

A diabetic diet is not only helpful for managing diabetes, but it also comes with many benefits as well. Eating a diet abundant in vegetables, fruits, and fiber can reduce your risk of heart disease and certain types of cancer.

Eating or drinking dairy products that are low in fat can reduce your chances of developing low bone mass in the future. Here is a list of great benefits that comes with eating a diabetic diet:

- ❖ Maintain general health
- ❖ Improve blood glucose control
- ❖ Obtain the desired blood lipid (fat) levels
- ❖ Maintain a normal blood pressure
- ❖ Keep a healthy body weight
- ❖ Stop or slow the progression of complications from diabetes

POSSIBLE RISKS

If you have diabetes, you must collaborate with your doctor and dietitian to develop a healthy eating plan that is perfect for you.

Make sure to stick to your diet so that you don't risk having fluctuating blood sugar levels or other serious complications. You can manage your diabetes as long as you control your blood glucose levels by eating healthy foods, watching your portion sizes, and planning ahead of time.

SAMPLE MEAL PLAN

When creating a meal plan, it's important to select foods that you will enjoy that will also fill you up. You don't want your diet to be a hindrance to you; instead, you want it to perfectly fit your preferences. You can control your blood glucose levels by including a small amount of carbohydrates in each meal or snack. Your main course can be served at either lunch or dinner.

Breakfast

Here are a few meals you can eat in the morning:

- ❖ ¾ –1 cup of high-fiber cereal, low-fat milk, and a fruit of your
- ❖ choice
- ❖ ½ cup of muesli or oats with low-fat milk or low-fat yogurt
- ❖ 2 slices of wholegrain toasted bread with peanut butter and a side
- ❖ of baked beans, boiled or poached eggs, or sardines
- ❖ Water, tea, or coffee

<u>Light Meal</u>

Some tasty light meals you can eat are:

- ❖ 1 sandwich made with slices of whole grain bread, or 6 small,
- ❖ high-fiber crackers and an avocado
- ❖ Salad
- ❖ 65–80g of lean meat or skinless poultry
- ❖ 100g of fish or other type of seafood
- ❖ 2 eggs or 1 cup of cooked legumes like beans or lentils
- ❖ Water, tea, or coffee

<u>Main Meal</u>

For your main meal you can have:

- ❖ ½ 1 cup cooked whole grain rice or pasta, or 1-2 small potatoes
- ❖ Other types of low-starch vegetables
- ❖ 65–80g of lean meat or skinless poultry
- ❖ 100g fish or other type of seafood
- ❖ 1 cup of cooked legumes like beans or lentils
- ❖ Water, tea, or coffee

<u>Between-Meal Snacks</u>

Snacks are tasty! Choosing ones that are healthy for persons with diabetes is crucial. If you don't know whether or not a certain snack food is appropriate for your way of eating, you can consult your diabetes educator or a dietitian. Here are several healthy snacks you might like:

- ❖ Fresh fruits
- ❖ A bit of reduced-fat natural yogurt
- ❖ A glass of skim milk
- ❖ 1 piece of whole grain bread with peanut butter, ricotta or cottage cheese, and tomato
- ❖ 1 slice of fruit bread
- ❖ High-fiber crackers with the same toppings as the bread above

You should consult a dietitian about your eating habits so that appropriate dietary recommendations can be developed for your specific needs. You should also talk with your doctor to ensure that the diet plan you choose is the best for your body and your condition.

This book will undoubtedly assist you on your journey. While you may believe that being diabetic limits your food options to bland, healthy foods, we are here to prove you wrong. This book contains a variety of recipes that are not only delicious but also nutritious. It's ideal for those who are new to a diabetic diet, and we've included a healthy meal plan to help you stay on track. It's a great resource not only for those with diabetes or prediabetes but also for those who want to try living a healthier lifestyle.

DIABETES AND NUTRITION

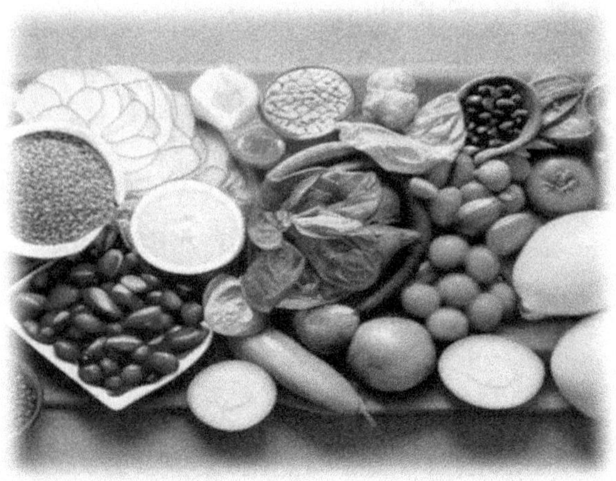

Today is the first day of your journey to good health and well-being with a top-notch diabetes nutrition plan. As you learned in the Introduction, the majority of diabetes care is self-care. Managing your nutrition when you have diabetes involves learning as much as you can about your condition as well as making positive behavior changes related to food. It's time to get started learning about diabetes and its relationship to food.

Even if you've just been diagnosed with type 2 diabetes, you may be surprised to find that you could have had diabetes for quite some time. This is because type 2 diabetes usually develops gradually, and its symptoms can be so subtle that they may go unnoticed for a while. Looking back, you might realize that you had some of these classic diabetes symptoms even before you were diagnosed:

- Urinating frequently
- Feeling really thirsty
- Feeling incredibly hungry
- Unusual tiredness
- Blurry vision
- Cuts and bruises that are sluggish to heal
- Unexplained weight loss
- Tingling, discomfort, or numbness in your hands or feet
- Dry or itching skin
- Recurring infections

Many individuals ignore these symptoms or just put them up to "getting older." Then they put off visiting their health-care provider because the symptoms don't appear significant, which further delays the diabetes diagnosis. If you have already been diagnosed with type 2 diabetes, then you may know that your family might possibly have a higher risk for the ailment. Fortunately, the same healthy eating and physical activity regimen that you will be following may provide your family members a greater chance at postponing or avoiding type 2 diabetes if they accompany you in your path toward health and well-being.

Can Diabetes Be Prevented?

Type 2 diabetes is a lifelong illness indicated by excessive levels of glucose (sugar) in the blood. It starts when the body does not react adequately to insulin, which is a hormone secreted by the pancreas. Insulin enables glucose to travel into cells, so the glucose may be utilized for energy. If glucose doesn't get into the cells, then it will build up in the circulation, causing the signs of diabetes.

Insulin resistance and obesity are generally linked with type 2 diabetes. Insulin resistance implies that adipose, liver, and muscle cells do not react appropriately to insulin, and, as a consequence, the pancreas generates more and more insulin. But over time it isn't able to keep up. Eventually, the pancreas cannot generate enough insulin to match the higher requirements, and then blood glucose levels increase. The diagnosis of prediabetes or diabetes is depending on the findings of blood glucose tests. (More information about prediabetes follows.)

Type 2 diabetes is a progressive illness that develops in a predictable pattern. Over time, the body's insulin-producing cells progressively lose their capacity to work efficiently, and therapies such as oral medicines, injectable medicines, or both may be needed—in addition to proper nutrition, active exercise, and habit change—to maintain the optimal blood glucose management.

The good news is that the progressive nature of type 2 diabetes typically helps you or your health-care practitioner to spot the development disease in its early stage, termed as prediabetes. Making simple living modifications at the site of prediabetes may prevent or postpone the development of type 2 diabetes.

THE WHOLE BODY EFFECT

Diabetes, unlike virtually any other known illness, has the unique and cancerous capacity to damage our whole body. Practically no organ system stays unaltered by diabetes. These complications

are often characterized as either microvascular (small blood vessels) or macro vascular (large blood vessels). Certain organs, such as the eyes, kidneys, and nerves, are largely supplied by tiny blood arteries. Damage to these little blood vessels resulting in the visual issues, chronic renal disease, and nerve damage often observed in people with long-standing diabetes. Collectively, they are termed microvascular illnesses. Other organs, such as the heart, brain, and legs, are perfused by big blood vessels. Damage to bigger blood vessels occurs in narrowing termed atherosclerotic plaque. When this plaque ruptures, it promotes the inflammation and blood clots that cause heart attacks, strokes, and gangrene of the legs. Together, they are known as macro vascular disorders.

How diabetes causes this damage to blood vessels will be covered throughout this book. It was usually regarded to be just a result of elevated blood glucose, but the fact, as we'll discover, is significantly different. Beyond the vascular disorders are numerous other concerns, including skin problems, fatty liver disease, infections, polycystic ovarian syndrome, Alzheimer's disease, and cancer. However, let's begin with the challenges linked with little blood vessels.

MICROVASCULAR COMPLICATIONS

Retinopathy

Diabetes is the primary cause of blindness in the United States. Eye disease—characteristically retinal degeneration (retinopathy)—is one of the most prevalent consequences of diabetes. The retina is the light sensitive nerve layer at the back of the eye that transmits its "picture" to the brain. Diabetes impairs the tiny, retinal blood vessels, which causes blood and other fluids to seep out. During normal physical eye exams, this leakage may be observed using a standard ophthalmoscope. In response to this injury, new retinal blood vessels grow, but they are delicate and easily broken. The outcome is increased bleeding and the eventual creation of scar tissue. In extreme circumstances, this scar tissue may elevate the retina and drag it away from its usual location, eventually leading to blindness. Laser therapy may prevent retinopathy by closing or eliminating the leaky young blood vessels. Approximately 10,000 new instances of blindness in the United States are caused by diabetic retinopathy per year.

Whether

Retinopathy develops relies on how long a person has had diabetes as well as how serious the condition is, in type 1 diabetes, most people get some degree of retinopathy within twenty years. In type 2 diabetes, retinopathy may really develop up to seven years before the diabetes itself is diagnosed.

Nephropathy

The main job of the kidneys is to clear the blood. When they fail, toxins build up in the body, which leads to lack of appetite, weight loss, and continuous nausea and vomiting. If the illness goes ignored, it ultimately leads to coma and death. In the United States, more than 100,000 people are diagnosed with chronic renal disease yearly, costing $32 billion in 2005. The burden is not only monetarily significant, but emotionally terrible.

Diabetic kidney disease (nephropathy) is the primary cause of end stage renal disease

(ESRD) in the United States, accounting for 44 percent of all new cases in 2005.

Patients whose kidneys have lost over 90 percent of their inherent function requiring dialysis to artificially eliminate the stored toxins in the blood. This technique entails taking the patient's "dirty" blood, running it via the dialysis machine to filter out its contaminants, and then restoring the clean blood to the body. To remain alive, patients need four hours of dialysis, three times each week, forever, unless they obtain a transplant. Diabetic kidney damage sometimes takes fifteen to twenty-five years to occur, although, like retinopathy, it may sometimes be identified before type 2 diabetes, itself. Approximately 2 percent of type 2 diabetes persons get renal damage each year. Ten years' after diagnosis, 25 percent of patients will show indications of renal disease.

Once established, diabetic nephropathy tends to develop, leading to further and more renal dysfunction till finally the patient needs dialysis or transplantation.

Neuropathy

Diabetic nerve damage (neuropathy) affects roughly 60–70 % of people with diabetes. Once again, the longer the length and severity of diabetes, the higher the risk of neuropathy.

There are several distinct forms of diabetic nerve injury. Commonly, diabetic neuropathy affects the peripheral nerves, initially in the feet, and then increasingly in the hands and arms as well, in a typical stocking-and-glove distribution. Damage to various kinds of nerves will result in varied symptoms, including;

- tingling,
- numbness,
- burning, and
- pain.

The continuous agony of severe diabetic neuropathy is devastating, and the symptoms are typically worst at night. Even powerful medicines such as narcotic drugs are generally useless. Instead of discomfort, individuals may occasionally feel full numbness. Careful physical examination indicates diminished feelings of touch, vibration, and temperature, and a lack of reflexes in the afflicted sections of the body. While a lack of feeling may appear benign, it is everything but. Pain shields us from detrimental trauma. When we stub our toes, we lay in the improper posture, discomfort informs us know that we should soon modify ourselves in order to avoid future tissue injury. If we are unable to sense pain, we may continue to undergo repeated instances of trauma. Over years, the damage becomes gradual and occasionally deformative. A simple example is the foot. Significant nerve injury might lead to the ultimate loss of the joint—a ailment termed Charcot foot—and may proceed to the point where people are unable to walk, and may possibly need amputation.

Another nerve condition affecting the big muscle groups is termed diabetic amyotrophy, which is characterized by intense discomfort and muscular weakness, notably in the thighs.

The autonomic nerve system governs our automatic body functions, including as breathing, digestion, sweating, and heart rate. Damage to these nerves may induce nausea, vomiting, constipation, diarrhea, bladder dysfunction, erectile dysfunction, and orthostatic hypotension (a quick, dramatic decrease in blood pressure on standing up). If the nerves to the heart are damaged, the risk of silent heart attacks and death increases. No existing medication restores diabetic nerve damage. Drugs may relieve the symptoms of the condition but do not modify its inherent history. Ultimately, it can only be avoided.

MACROVASCULAR COMPLICATIONS

Atherosclerosis (hardening of the arteries)

Atherosclerosis is a condition of the arteries wherein plaques of fatty particles are deposited into the inner walls of the blood vessel, producing narrowing and hardness. This condition causes heart attacks, strokes, and peripheral vascular disease, which are collectively termed as cardiovascular disorders. Diabetes significantly raises the chance of acquiring atherosclerosis.

Atherosclerosis is widely yet wrongly viewed as cholesterol progressively blocking the arteries, same as sludge could develop up in a pipe. In reality, it comes from damage to the artery, albeit the specific cause of the damage is uncertain. There are numerous relevant variables, including but not limited to age, genetics, smoking, diabetes, stress, high blood pressure, and lack of physical activity. Any break of the artery's walls might trigger an inflammatory cascade. Cholesterol (a waxy, fat-like substance present in all cells of the body) infiltrates the injured region and narrows the blood channel.

The smooth muscle that supports the tissue of the blood vessel proliferates, and collagen, a structural molecule presents abundantly in the body, also builds in reaction to this harm. Again, the outcome is a further constriction of the blood artery. Rather than a single event that may be quickly mended, this response happens in reply to persistent damage to the vessel wall. The final effect is the growth of plaque, known as the atheroma, which is a pocket of cholesterol, smooth muscle cells, and inflammatory cells within the blood vessel wall. This gradually restricts the flow of blood to damaged organs. If this atheroma ruptures, a blood clot develops. The abrupt occlusion of the artery by the clot hinders regular blood circulation and starves the downstream cells of oxygen, leading cell death and cardiovascular disease.

Heart Disease

heart attacks, known medically as myocardial infarctions, are the most well-recognized and dreaded consequence of diabetes. They are caused by atherosclerosis of the blood arteries feeding the heart. The unexpected occlusion of these arteries starves the heart of oxygen, resulting in the demise of part of the heart muscle. The Framingham studies in the 1970s demonstrated a strong link between cardiac disease and diabetes.

Diabetes raises the risk of cardiovascular disease two- to fourfold, and these difficulties emerge at an earlier age compared to nondiabetics. Sixty-eight percent of diabetics aged sixty-five or older will die of heart disease, and a further 16 percent will die of stroke. Reducing the risk of macrovascular disease is thus of main importance. The level of fatalities and disability stemming from cardiovascular illnesses is several times bigger than that resulting from microvascular disorders.

Over the last three decades, there have been substantial advancements in the treatment of cardiac disease, but gains for diabetic patients have fallen far behind. While the total mortality rate for nondiabetic males has reduced by 36.4 percent, it has only fell 13.1 percent for diabetic men.

Stroke

A stroke is induced by atherosclerosis of the major blood arteries supplying the brain. An unexpected disturbance of the normal blood flow starves the brain of oxygen and a section of the brain may die. Symptoms vary depending upon where section of the brain is damaged, however the terrible effect of stroke cannot be underestimated. In the United States, it is the third largest cause of mortality and the largest factor to disability.

Diabetes is a substantial independent risk factor in stroke, suggesting that, on its own, diabetes raises a person's chance of having a stroke by as much as 150–400 percent. Approximately a fourth of all new strokes occur in diabetic patients. Every year of diabetes raises the incidence of stroke by 3 percent, and the prognosis is also significantly worse.

Peripheral vascular disease

Peripheral Vascular Disease (PVD) is caused by atherosclerosis of the big blood vessels feeding the legs. The disturbance of normal blood flow starves the legs of oxygen-carrying hemoglobin. The most typical sign of PVD is discomfort or cramping that develops with walking and is eased by rest. As the blood vessels constrict and circulation worsens, discomfort may sometimes emerge during rest and particularly at night. PVD substantially decreases mobility, which might lead to long-term disability. Skin with a weak blood supply is more likely to be injured and takes longer to recover. In diabetics, small cuts or injuries to the foot may develop non-healing foot ulcers. In extreme circumstances, these places where the skin has broken away, exposing underlying tissue, may proceed to gangrene. At this moment, blood supply has been considerably diminished or entirely lost, the tissue dies, and amputation of the damaged limb—a therapy of last resort—often becomes required help cure persistent infections and reduce pain.

Diabetes, along with smoking, is the biggest risk factor for PVD. Approximately 27 percent of diabetic people with PVD will steadily deteriorate during a five-year period, and 4 percent of them will necessitate an amputation.17 Patients with gangrene and those needing amputation may never walk again, which might result in a cycle of infirmity. A decrease of function of the limbs leads to less physical exercise, which in turn leads to gradual deconditioning of the muscles. Weaker muscles lead to less physical activity, and the cycle repeats.

OTHER COMPLICATIONS

Alzheimer's disease

Alzheimer's Disease is a chronic, progressive, neurodegenerative sickness that causes memory loss, personality problems, and cognitive issues. It is the most prevalent kind of dementia, and the sixth greatest cause of mortality in the United States.18 Alzheimer's illness may signify the inability to utilize glucose properly, potentially a form of specific insulin resistance in the brain. The ties between Alzheimer's disease and diabetes have gotten so powerful that many researchers have indicated Alzheimer's disease might be designated type 3 diabetes. These points go much beyond the scope of this work, however.

Cancer

Type 2 diabetes raises the risk of most prevalent malignancies, including breast, stomach, colorectal, kidney, and endometrial malignancies. This may be connected to some of the drugs used to treat diabetes It will be further covered in chapter 10. The survival rate of cancer patients with pre-existing diabetes is considerably worse than for nondiabetics.

Fatty liver disease

Non-Alcoholic Fatty liver disease (NAFLD) is described as the storing The buildup of extra fat in the form of triglycerides surpassing 5 percent of the total weight of the liver. This condition can be found utilizing an ultrasound to scan the abdomen. When this excess fat causes damage to the liver tissue, which may be revealed Using normal blood testing, it is labeled non-alcoholic steato-hepatitis (NASH). Current estimates imply that NAFLD affects 30 percent and NASH 5 percent of the U.S. population; both are primary causes of hepatic cirrhosis (irreversible scarring of the liver).

NAFLD is almost non-existent in recent-onset type 1 diabetes. By Conversely, the incidence of type 2 diabetes is estimated at upwards of 75 percent. The key significance of fatty liver is more extensively addressed in

Infections

Diabetics are more prone to all forms of illnesses, which are triggered by alien organisms infiltrating and proliferating in the body. Not only are they more sensitive to various forms of bacterial and fungal infections than nondiabetics, the consequences also likely to be greater serious. For example, diabetics have a four- to fivefold increased chance of causing a significant kidney infection. All forms of fungal infections, include thrush, vaginal yeast infections, fungal infections of the nails, and athlete's foot, are more frequent in diabetes people.

Among the most dangerous illnesses for diabetes are those affecting the feet. Despite good blood glucose management, 15 % of all diabetes individuals will suffer non-healing foot wounds throughout their lifespan. Infections in these wounds typically involve many bacteria, making broad-spectrum antibiotic therapy necessary. However, the reduced blood circulation associated with PVD (see above) adds to the poor wound healing. As a consequence, diabetics have a fifteen-fold greater risk of lower-limb amputation, and account for nearly 50 percent of the amputations done in the United States, excluding accidents. It is estimated that each of these instances of infected diabetic foot ulcers costs upwards of $25,000 to treat.

There are several contributing variables to the increased rates of infection. High blood glucose may damage the immune system. As well, inadequate blood circulation lowers the effectiveness of infection-fighting white blood cells to reach all regions of the body.

Skin and nail conditions

Numerous skin and nail problems are connected to diabetes. Generally, they are more of a cosmetic problem than a medical one; yet, they frequently reflect the underlying dangerous disease of diabetes, which needs medical management. Acanthosis nigricans is a gray-black, velvety thickening of the skin, especially around the neck and in body folds, induced by high insulin levels. Diabetic dermopathy, sometimes termed shin spots, are typically seen on the lower limbs as black, coarsely scaled lesions. Skin tags are delicate protrusions of skin typically present on the eyelids, neck, and

armpits. Over 25 percent of people with skin tags have diabetes.

Nail issues are very frequent in diabetes people, particularly fungal infections. The nails may grow yellowy-brown, thicken, and detach from the nail bed (onycholysis).

Erectile dysfunction

Community-Based Population study of men aged 39–70 years found indicates the prevalence of impotence varies between 10 and 50 percent. Diabetes is a critical risk factor, raising the likelihood of erectile malfunctioning more than tenfold and impacting patients at a younger age than typical. Poor blood circulation in diabetics is the probable explanation for this higher risk. The incidence of erectile dysfunction also rises increased age and degree of insulin resistance, with an estimated 50-60 percent of diabetic males over the age of 50 experiencing this problem.

Polycystic ovarian syndrome

An imbalance of the hormones may cause some women to develop cysts (benign lumps) on the ovaries. This condition, termed polycystic ovarian syndrome (PCOS), is characterized by irregular menstrual cycles, signs of excessive testosterone, and the presence of cysts (typically found by ultrasound). PCOS sufferers have many of the same features as type 2 diabetics, including obesity, high blood pressure, high cholesterol, and insulin resistance. PCOS is characterized by high insulin resistance26 and raises the risk of acquiring type 2 diabetes three-to fivefold in young women.

TREAT THE CAUSE, NOT THE SYMPTOMS

Whereas most diseases are restricted to a specific organ system, diabetes impacts every organ in many ways. As a consequence, it is the leading cause of blindness. It is the major cause of renal failure. It is the main cause of heart disease. It is the leading cause of stroke. It is the primary cause of amputations. It is the primary cause of dementia. It is the major cause of infertility. It is the primary cause of nerve injury. But the confusing issue is why these difficulties are increasing worse, not better, even years after the illness was initially described. As our knowledge of diabetes advances, we anticipate that complications should reduce. But they don't. If the situation is becoming worse, then the only reasonable explanation is that our understanding and treatment of type 2 diabetes is fundamentally flawed. We concentrate relentlessly on reducing blood glucose. But high blood glucose is merely the symptom, not the reason. The fundamental cause of the hyperglycemia in type 2 diabetes is significant insulin resistance. Until we address that fundamental cause, insulin resistance, the pandemic of type 2 diabetes and all of its accompanying consequences will continue to get worse.

We need to start over. What causes type 2 diabetes? What causes insulin resistance and how can we reverse it? Obviously, obesity has a big influence. We must begin with the aetiology of obesity.

Reciepe Card

INGREDIENTS

INSTRUCTIONS

Serves

Prep

Cook Time

TIPS & TRICKS

NOTES

30-DAYS MEAL PLAN

This plan features breakfast, lunch, dinner, and snack options for each day, with occasional dessert suggestions. All recipes are mindful of diabetic dietary needs and are low in carbohydrates and sugar. Remember to adjust portion sizes based on your individual needs

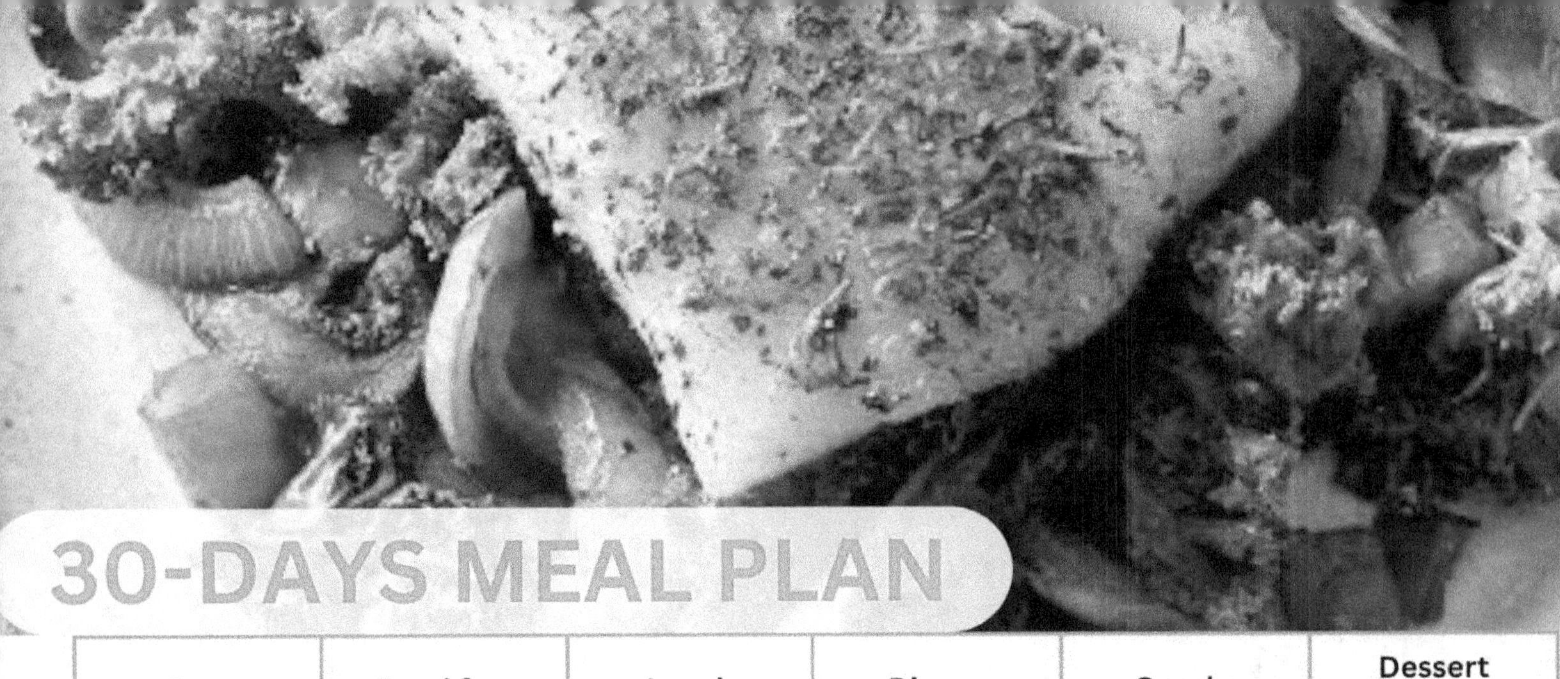

30-DAYS MEAL PLAN

Day	Breakfast	Lunch	Dinner	Snacks	Dessert (Optional)
1	Scrambled Eggs with Spinach & Tomatoes	Leftover Chicken & Vegetable Penne with Parsley-Walnut Pesto	Grilled Tilapia with Hazelnut-Parsley Roast & Brown Rice	Strawberry & Mango Smoothie	No-Bake Chocolate Cheesecake
2	Greek Yogurt with Berries & Chopped Almonds	Tuna Salad with Lettuce Wraps & Avocado Slices	Charred Vegetable & Bean Tostadas with Lime Crema	Cantaloupe Smoothie	Raspberry & Mango Smoothie
3	Whole-Wheat Toast with Cottage Cheese & Fruit	Leftover Grilled Tilapia with Hazelnut-Parsley Roast & Salad	Chicken & Vegetable Stir-Fry with Brown Rice	Berry & Spinach Smoothie	Pumpkin & Banana Ice Cream
4	Omelette with Bell Peppers & Onions	Turkey and Avocado Salad Sandwich on Whole-Wheat Bread	Shrimp Scampi with Zucchini Noodles	Hard-boiled egg with cucumber slices	Brulee Oranges
5	Peanut Butter Oatmeal with Chia Seeds	Leftover Chicken & Vegetable Stir-Fry	Roasted Salmon with Brussels Sprouts & Lemon Butter	Cottage cheese with pineapple chunks	No-Bake Chocolate Cheesecake
6	Chia Seed Pudding with Berries	Beef Lettuce Wraps with Asian-Style Dressing	Turkey Meatloaf with Sweet Potato Mash	Edamame pods with sprinkled chili flakes	Frozen Blueberry Lemondae
7	Scrambled Eggs with Smoked Salmon & Asparagus	Leftover Turkey Meatloaf with Mixed Greens Salad	Black Bean Burgers on Whole-Wheat Buns with Sweet Potato Fries	Greek yogurt with cinnamon and chopped nuts	Easy Keto Chocolate Mousse
8	Whole-Wheat Toast with Avocado & Sliced Tomato	Salmon Salad Sandwich on Rye Bread	Lentil Soup with Whole-Wheat Bread	Carrot sticks with hummus	Keto Tiramisu

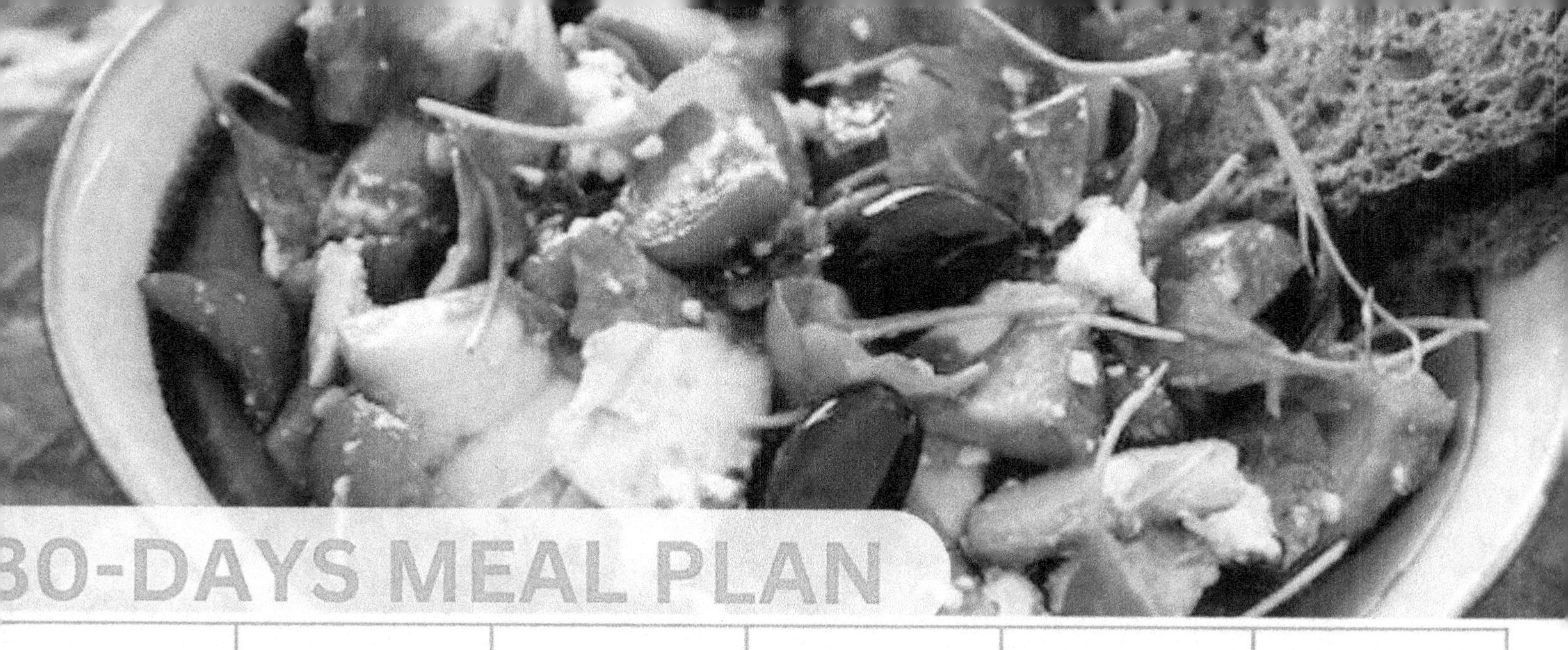

9	Greek Yogurt with Berries & Granola	Leftover Lentil Soup & Salad	One-Pan Roasted Chicken with Vegetables	Celery sticks with almond butter	Keto Chocolate Avocado Mousse
10	Baked Eggs with Spinach & Feta	Turkey & Cheese Roll-Ups	Shrimp & Veggie Kebabs with Brown Rice	Apple slices with almond butter	Keto Lemon Bars
11	Cottage Cheese with Fruit & Chia Seeds	Chicken Salad with Lettuce Wraps	Baked Cod with Lemon & Herbs	Edamame pods with sea salt	Pumpkin & Spice Smoothie
12	Omelette with Mushrooms & Swiss Cheese	Tuna Salad with Whole-Wheat Crackers	Veggie Burgers on Whole-Wheat Buns with Avocado	Cucumber slices with yogurt dip	Strawberry & Mango Smoothie
13	Peanut Butter Banana Toast	Leftover Veggie Burgers & Salad	Turkey Chili with Kidney Beans & Brown Rice	Carrot sticks with ranch dressing	No-Bake Chocolate Cheesecake
14	Whole-Wheat Pancakes with Berries & Yogurt	Tuna & Veggie Wraps	Salmon with Roasted Asparagus & Quinoa	Bell pepper slices with guacamole	Frozen Blueberry Lemondae
15	Scrambled Eggs with Smoked Salmon & Capers	Leftover Salmon & Roasted Asparagus	Chicken Stir-Fry with Broccoli & Brown Rice	Cottage cheese with pineapple chunks	Easy Keto Chocolate Mousse
16	Cottage Cheese with Fruit & Nuts	Lentil Soup with Whole-Wheat Bread	Black Bean & Corn Salad with Avocado	Celery sticks with peanut butter	Keto Tiramisu

30-DAYS MEAL PLAN

17	Omelette with Bell Peppers & Onions	Leftover Black Bean & Corn Salad	Turkey Meatloaf with Sweet Potato Mash	Apple slices with almond butter	Keto Chocolate Avocado Mousse
18	Greek Yogurt with Berries & Granola	Tuna Salad Sandwich on Rye Bread	Shrimp Scampi with Zucchini Noodles	Edamame pods with sea salt	Pumpkin & Spice Smoothie
19	Chia Seed Pudding with Berries	Leftover Shrimp Scampi & Salad	One-Pan Roasted Chicken with Vegetables	Carrot sticks with hummus	Keto Lemon Bars
20	Baked Eggs with Spinach & Feta	Turkey & Cheese Roll-Ups	Chicken & Veggie Stir-Fry with Brown Rice	Celery sticks with almond butter	Frozen Blueberry Lemondae
21	Whole-Wheat Toast with Avocado & Sliced Tomato	Leftover Chicken & Veggie Stir-Fry	Salmon with Roasted Asparagus & Quinoa	Cucumber slices with yogurt dip	No-Bake Chocolate Cheesecake
22	Cottage Cheese with Fruit & Chia Seeds	Tuna Salad with Lettuce Wraps	Black Bean Burgers on Whole-Wheat Buns with Avocado	Apple slices with almond butter	Easy Keto Chocolate Mousse
23	Omelette with Mushrooms & Swiss Cheese	Leftover Black Bean Burgers & Salad	Turkey Chili with Kidney Beans & Brown Rice	Carrot sticks with ranch dressing	No-Bake Chocolate Cheesecake

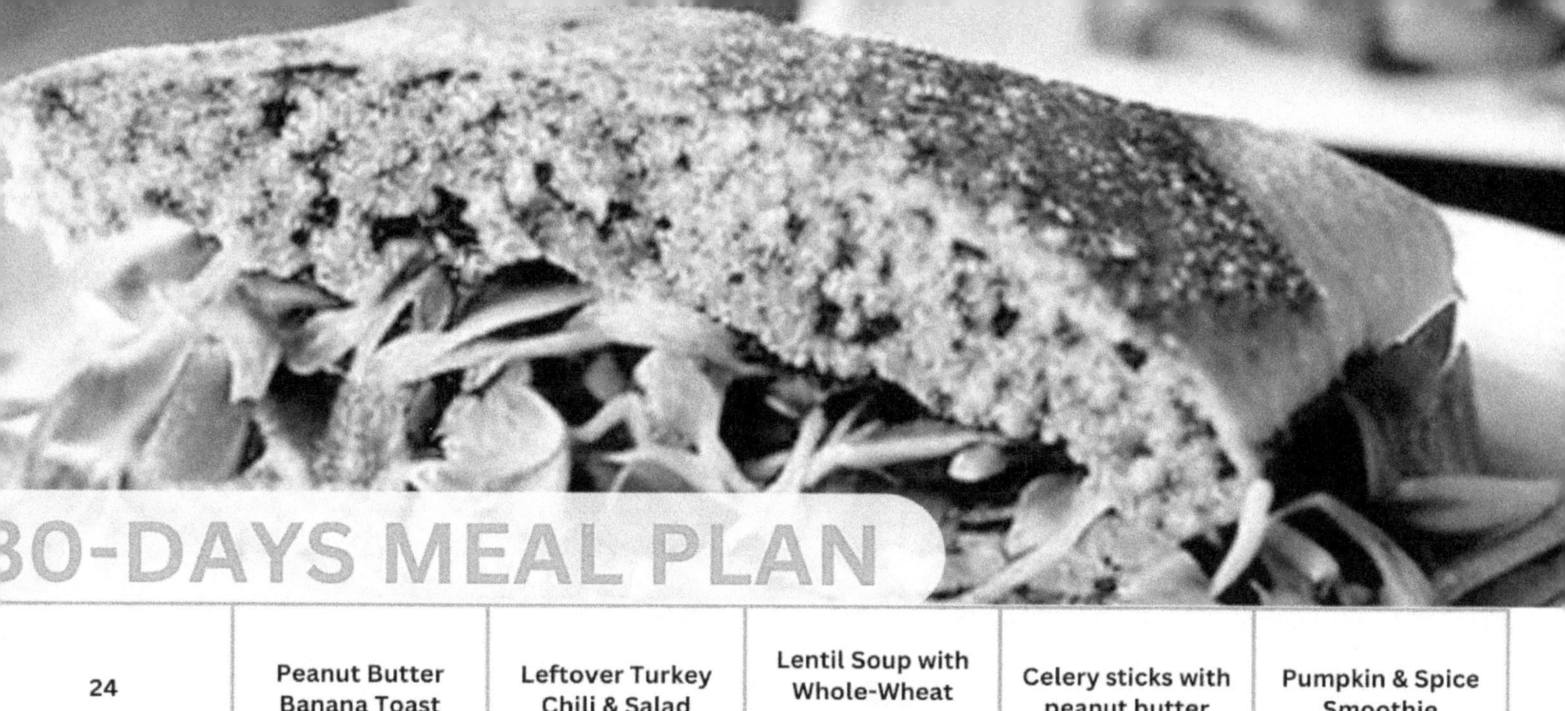

24	Peanut Butter Banana Toast	Leftover Turkey Chili & Salad	Lentil Soup with Whole-Wheat Bread	Celery sticks with peanut butter	Pumpkin & Spice Smoothie
25	Whole-Wheat Pancakes with Berries & Yogurt	Tuna & Veggie Wraps	Salmon with Roasted Asparagus & Quinoa	Bell pepper slices with guacamole	Keto Tiramisu
26	Scrambled Eggs with Smoked Salmon & Capers	Leftover Salmon & Roasted Asparagus	Chicken Stir-Fry with Broccoli & Brown Rice	Cottage cheese with pineapple chunks	Easy Keto Chocolate Mousse
27	Greek Yogurt with Berries & Granola	Leftover Chicken Stir-Fry	One-Pan Roasted Chicken with Vegetables	Apple slices with almond butter	Brulee Oranges
28	Chia Seed Pudding with Berries	Leftover One-Pan Roasted Chicken & Salad	Shrimp Scampi with Zucchini Noodles	Edamame pods with sea salt	Frozen Blueberry Lemondae
29	Baked Eggs with Spinach & Feta	Turkey & Cheese Roll-Ups	Chicken & Veggie Stir-Fry with Brown Rice	Celery sticks with hummus	No-Bake Chocolate Cheesecake
30	Whole-Wheat Toast with Avocado & Sliced Tomato	Leftover Chicken & Veggie Stir-Fry	Salmon with Roasted Asparagus & Quinoa	Cucumber slices with yogurt dip	Keto Strawberry Shortcake

Reciepe Card

INGREDIENTS

INSTRUCTIONS

TIPS & TRICKS

NOTES

BREAKFAST QUESADILLA

- **Prep Time: 5 minutes**
- **Serving Time: 2 minutes**
- **Cooking Time: 10 minutes**

NUTRITIONAL VALUE (PER SERVING):

- Calories: 350
- Fat: 15g
- Saturated Fat: 7g
- Carbohydrates: 30g
- Fiber: 3g
- Sugar: 2g
- Protein: 15g

INGREDIENTS:

- 1 big flour tortilla
- ¼ cup shredded cheddar cheese
- 2 big eggs, scrambled
- 2 slices cooked bacon

INSTRUCTIONS:

1. Heat a large skillet over medium heat.
2. Spread cheese evenly over one side of the tortilla.
3. Top with scrambled eggs and bacon.
4. Fold the tortilla in half.
5. Cook for 2-3 minutes each side, or until golden brown and cheese has melted.
6. Cut into wedges and serve with your favorite salsa or spicy sauce.

Tip:

- For a fuller quesadilla, add some cooked black beans or veggies.

Serving Suggestion: Serve with a side of fruit or yogurt for a full breakfast.

REDUCED CARB BERRY PARFAITS

- **Prep Time: 10 minutes**
- **Serving Time: 2 minutes**
- **Cooking Time: 0 minutes**

NUTRITIONAL VALUE (PER SERVING):

- Calories: 250
- Fat: 10g
- Saturated Fat: 5g
- Carbohydrates: 30g
- Fiber: 5g
- Sugar: 10g
- Protein: 10g

INGREDIENTS:

- ½ cup plain Greek yogurt

- ¼ cup mixed berries
- 1 tablespoon chopped nuts 1 tablespoon powdered flaxseed

INSTRUCTIONS:

1. Layer yogurt, berries, almonds, and flaxseed in a parfait glass.

Tip:

- For a sweeter parfait, add a drizzle of honey or maple syrup.

Serving Suggestion: Enjoy this parfait as a quick and simple breakfast or snack.

HEALTHY AVOCADO TOAST

- **Prep Time: 5 minutes**
- **Serving Time: 2 minutes**
- **Cooking Time: 0 minutes**

NUTRITIONAL VALUE (PER SERVING):

- Calories: 350
- Fat: 20g
- Saturated Fat: 4g
- Carbohydrates: 35g
- Fiber: 5g
- Sugar: 1g
- Protein: 8g

INGREDIENTS:

- 1-piece whole-wheat bread
- ½ avocado, mashed
- 1 tablespoon chopped tomato
- 1 tablespoon crumbled feta cheese
- A teaspoon of salt and pepper to taste

INSTRUCTIONS:

- Toast the bread.
- Spread avocado on the bread.
- Top with tomato, feta cheese, salt, and pepper.

Tip:

- For more savory toast, add a dab of olive oil or balsamic vinegar.

Serving Suggestion: Serve this toast as a quick and simple breakfast or snack.

ZUCCHINI BREAD PANCAKES

- **Prep Time: 15 minutes**
- **Serving Time: 5 minutes**
- **Cooking Time: 10 minutes**

NUTRITIONAL VALUE (PER SERVING):

- Calories: 250
- Fat: 10g
- Saturated Fat: 2g
- Carbohydrates: 30g
- Fiber: 4g
- Sugar: 5g
- Protein: 8g

INGREDIENTS:

- 1 cup grated zucchini
- ½ cup whole-wheat flour ¼ cup unsweetened applesauce
- 2 eggs
- 1 tablespoon honey
- 1 teaspoon baking powder
- ½ teaspoon baking soda
- ¼ teaspoon cinnamon
- A pinch of salt

INSTRUCTIONS:

- Preheat oven to 350 degrees F (175 degrees C).
- In a large basin, mix zucchini, flour, applesauce, eggs, honey, baking powder, baking soda, cinnamon, and salt.
- Heat a large skillet over medium heat and oil with butter or cooking spray.
- Drop ¼-cupfuls of batter into the skillet and cook for 2-3 minutes each side, or until golden brown.
- Transfer pancakes to a baking sheet and bake for 5-10 minutes, or until cooked through.
- Serve warm with maple syrup and fruit.

Tip:

- For a more luxurious breakfast, top pancakes with whipped cream and a sprinkling of cinnamon.

RED PEPPER, GOAT CHEESE, AND ARUGULA OPEN-FACED GRILLED SANDWICH

- **Prep Time: 10 minutes**
- **Serving Time: 2 minutes**
- **Cooking Time: 5 minutes**

NUTRITIONAL VALUE (PER SERVING):

- Calories: 300
- Fat: 15g
- Saturated Fat: 5g
- Carbohydrates: 25g
- Fiber: 3g
- Sugar: 2g
- Protein: 10g

INGREDIENTS:

- 1-piece whole-wheat bread
- ¼ cup roasted red peppers
- 2 ounces' goat cheese
- 1 cup arugula
- A sprinkle of olive oil
- Salt and pepper to taste

INSTRUCTIONS:

- Preheat a grill pan or panini press over medium heat.

- Spread goat cheese on the toast.
- Top with roasted red peppers and arugula.
- Drizzle with olive oil.
- Grill for 2-3 minutes each side, or until bread is toasted and goat cheese is melted.
- Season with salt and pepper to taste.
- Serve warm.

Tip:

- For more savory sandwich, add a sprinkle of balsamic vinegar or red pepper flakes.

WHOLE EGG BAKED SWEET POTATOES

- **Prep Time: 10 minutes**
- **Serving Time: 2 minutes**
- **Cooking Time: 45 minutes**

NUTRITIONAL VALUE (PER SERVING):

- Calories: 400
- Fat: 10g
- Saturated Fat: 2g
- Carbohydrates: 60g
- Fiber: 6g
- Sugar: 40g
- Protein: 15g

INGREDIENTS:

- 1 medium sweet potato
- 1 tablespoon olive oil
- A sprinkle of salt and pepper

INSTRUCTIONS:

1. Preheat oven to 400 degrees F (200 degrees C).
2. Pierce the sweet potato with a fork many times.
3. Rub the sweet potato with olive oil.
4. Season with salt and pepper.
5. Place the sweet potato on a baking pan and bake for 45 minutes, or until soft.
6. Cut the sweet potato in half and scrape out the meat.
7. Mash the sweet potato with a fork.
8. Serve warm with your favorite toppings, such as cinnamon, maple syrup, or chopped nuts.

Tip:

- For a more delicious meal, add a dash of nutmeg or ginger.

BERRY AVOCADO SMOOTHIE

- **Prep Time: 5 minutes**
- **Serving Time: 1 minute**
- **Cooking Time: 0 minutes**

NUTRITIONAL VALUE (PER SERVING):

- Calories: 300
- Fat: 15g
- Saturated Fat: 3g
- Carbohydrates: 35g
- Fiber: 5g
- Sugar: 10g
- Protein: 5g

INGREDIENTS:

- ½ cup mixed berries
- ½ avocado
- 1 cup plain Greek yogurt
- ½ cup unsweetened almond milk
- 1 tablespoon honey

INSTRUCTIONS:

1. Combine all ingredients in a blender and mix until smooth.
2. Serve immediately.

Tip:

- For a thicker smoothie, add extra yogurt or almond milk. For a thinner smoothie, add extra water or ice.

BAGEL HUMMUS TOAST

- **Prep Time: 5 minutes**
- **Serving Time: 2 minutes**
- **Cooking Time: 0 minutes**

NUTRITIONAL VALUE (PER SERVING):

- Calories: 350

- Fat: 15g
- Saturated Fat: 3g
- Carbohydrates: 45g
- Fiber: 5g
- Sugar: 3g
- Protein: 10g

INGREDIENTS:

- 1 whole-wheat bagel, toasted ¼ cup hummus
- 2 sliced tomatoes
- 1 tablespoon chopped cucumbers
- A sprinkling of red pepper flakes

INSTRUCTIONS:

1. Spread hummus on the bagel.
2. Top with tomatoes, cucumbers, and red pepper flakes.
3. Serve immediately.

Tip:

- For more savory toast, add a dab of olive oil or balsamic vinegar.

BLACK BEAN TACOS BREAKFAST

- **Prep Time: 10 minutes**
- **Serving Time: 3 minutes**
- **Cooking Time: 10 minutes**

NUTRITIONAL VALUE (PER SERVING):

- Calories: 350
- Fat: 15g
- Saturated Fat: 3g
- Carbohydrates: 40g
- Fiber: 5g
- Sugar: 3g
- Protein: 10g

INGREDIENTS:

- 1 (15-ounce) can black beans, washed and drained
- 1 tablespoon olive oil
- ½ cup chopped red onion 1 clove garlic, minced
- 1 teaspoon ground cumin
- ½ teaspoon chili powder
- ¼ teaspoon salt ¼ teaspoon black pepper
- 1 tablespoon lime juice
- 4 warm corn tortillas
- ¼ cup chopped avocado
- ¼ cup chopped cilantro
- ¼ cup salsa

INSTRUCTIONS:

1. Heat the olive oil in a large pan over medium heat.
2. Add the onion and garlic and simmer until softened, approximately 5 minutes.
3. Stir in the black beans, cumin, chili powder, salt, and pepper.
4. Cook until the beans are cooked through, approximately 5 minutes.
5. Stir in the lime juice.
6. Warm the tortillas in a dry skillet or microwave for a few seconds.
7. Divide the bean mixture among the tortillas.
8. Top with avocado, cilantro, and salsa.

Tip:

- For a deeper taste, use mashed avocado instead of diced avocado.

Serving Suggestion: Serve with a side of fruit or yogurt for a full breakfast.

STRAWBERRY COCONUT BAKE

- **Prep Time: 15 minutes**
- **Serving Time: 2 minutes**
- **Cooking Time: 30 minutes**

NUTRITIONAL VALUE (PER SERVING):

- Calories: 400
- Fat: 20g
- Saturated Fat: 12g
- Carbohydrates: 50g
- Fiber: 4g
- Sugar: 25g
- Protein: 4g

INGREDIENTS:

- 1 cup all-purpose flour
- 1 cup unsweetened shredded coconut
- ½ cup granulated sugar
- ½ teaspoon baking powder
- ¼ teaspoon salt 1 cup diced fresh strawberries
- ½ cup unsweetened almond milk
- ¼ cup vegetable oil
- 1 teaspoon vanilla extract

INSTRUCTIONS:

1. Preheat oven to 350 degrees F (175 degrees C).
2. Grease a 9x13-inch baking dish.
3. In a large bowl, mix together flour, coconut, sugar, baking powder, and salt.
4. Stir in strawberries, almond milk, vegetable oil, and vanilla extract.
5. Pour batter into the prepared baking dish.
6. Bake for 30 minutes, or until golden brown and a toothpick inserted into the middle comes out clean.
7. Let cool slightly before serving.

Tip:

- For a more luxurious dessert, top with whipped cream and fresh strawberries.

PALEO BREAKFAST HASH

- **Prep Time: 10 minutes**
- **Serving Time: 3 minutes**
- **Cooking Time: 15 minutes**

NUTRITIONAL VALUE (PER SERVING):

- Calories: 400
- Fat: 20g
- Saturated Fat: 5g
- Carbohydrates: 35g
- Fiber: 5g
- Sugar: 5g
- Protein: 15g

INGREDIENTS:

- 1 tablespoon olive oil
- 1 medium sweet potato, peeled and chopped
- 1 medium onion, diced 1 green bell pepper, diced 1 red bell pepper, diced
- 1 (15-ounce) can chopped tomatoes, undrained
- 1 tablespoon chopped fresh parsley
- 1 teaspoon dried oregano
- ½ teaspoon salt ¼ teaspoon black pepper
- 4 big eggs

INSTRUCTIONS:

1. Heat the olive oil in a large pan over medium heat.

2. Add the sweet potato, onion, and bell peppers and simmer until softened, approximately 10 minutes.

3. Drain the chopped tomatoes, keeping the liquid.

4. Add the diced tomatoes, parsley, oregano, salt, and pepper to the skillet.

5. Cook for 5 minutes, stirring periodically.

6. Make 4 wells in the hash mixture.

7. Crack an egg into each well.

8. Cover the pan and heat until the egg whites are set, approximately 5 minutes.

9. Serve immediately.

Tip:

- For a deeper taste, add crumbled sausage or bacon instead of eggs.

OMELET WITH CHICKPEA FLOUR

- **Prep Time: 5 minutes**
- **Serving Time: 3 minutes**
- **Cooking Time: 10 minutes**

NUTRITIONAL VALUE (PER SERVING):

- Calories: 300
- Fat: 10g
- Saturated Fat: 2g
- Carbohydrates: 30g
- Fiber: 5g
- Sugar: 2g
- Protein: 15g

INGREDIENTS:

- ¼ cup chickpea flour
- 1 tablespoon olive oil
- 2 big eggs
- 1 tablespoon chopped veggies, such as spinach, mushrooms, or onions
- 1 tablespoon shredded cheese
- Salt and pepper to taste

INSTRUCTIONS:

1. In a small bowl, mix together chickpea flour and water until smooth.

2. Heat the olive oil in a nonstick skillet over medium heat.

3. Pour the chickpea flour batter into the pan and heat for 2-3 minutes, or until set.

4. Flip the omelet and cook for 2-3 minutes longer.

5. Add eggs, veggies, and cheese to the omelet.

6. Fold the omelet in half and cook until the eggs are set and the cheese is melted.

7. Season with salt and pepper to taste.

8. Serve immediately.

Tip:

- For tastier omelet, add your favorite herbs or spices.

TOAST WITH EGG AND AVOCADO

- Prep Time: 5 minutes
- Serving Time: 2 minutes
- Cooking Time: 5 minutes

NUTRITIONAL VALUE (PER SERVING):

- Calories: 350
- Fat: 20g
- Saturated Fat: 5g
- Carbohydrates: 35g
- Fiber: 5g
- Sugar: 1g
- Protein: 10g

INGREDIENTS:

- 1-piece whole-wheat bread
- 1 big egg
- ½ avocado, mashed
- A sprinkle of olive oil
- Salt and pepper to taste

INSTRUCTIONS:

1. Toast the bread.
2. In a small pan, heat the olive oil over medium heat.
3. Crack the egg into the skillet and heat until the whites are set and the yolks are cooked to your preference.
4. Spread avocado on the bread.
5. Top with the cooked egg.
6. Season with salt and pepper to taste.
7. Serve immediately.

Tip:

- For more savory toast, add a sprinkle of red pepper flakes or spicy sauce.

HUEVOS RANCHEROS

- Prep Time: 15 minutes
- Serving Time: 3 minutes
- Cooking Time: 10 minutes

NUTRITIONAL VALUE (PER SERVING):

- Calories: 450
- Fat: 25g
- Saturated Fat: 10g
- Carbohydrates: 30g

INGREDIENTS:

- 4 corn tortillas
- 1 (14.5-ounce) can chopped tomatoes, undrained
- 1 tablespoon olive oil
- 1 onion, chopped
- 1 jalapeño pepper, minced (optional)

- 1 clove garlic, minced
- 1 teaspoon chili powder
- ½ teaspoon ground cumin ¼ teaspoon salt ¼ teaspoon black pepper
- 4 big eggs

INSTRUCTIONS:

1. Warm the tortillas in a dry skillet or microwave for a few seconds.
2. In a medium saucepan, mix the chopped tomatoes, olive oil, onion, jalapeño pepper (if using), garlic, chili powder, cumin, salt, and pepper.
3. Bring to a boil and cook for 10 minutes, or until the sauce has thickened somewhat.
4. Fry the eggs in a separate pan over medium heat until done to your preference.
5. Place a tortilla on each platter.
6. Top with a dollop of salsa and a fried egg.
7. Serve immediately.

Tip:

- For a deeper taste, use homemade salsa instead of bottled salsa.

APPLE WALNUT FRENCH TOAST

- **Prep Time: 15 minutes**
- **Serving Time: 10 minutes**
- **Cooking Time: 10 minutes**

NUTRITIONAL VALUE (PER SERVING):

- Calories: 450
- Fat: 20g
- Saturated Fat: 5g
- Carbohydrates: 45g
- Fiber: 5g
- Sugar: 20g
- Protein: 12g

INGREDIENTS:

- 4 pieces of thick-cut challah bread
- 2 big eggs
- 1/2 cup milk
- 1 teaspoon vanilla extract
- 1/4 teaspoon ground cinnamon
- A pinch of salt
- 2 tablespoons butter
- 2 big apples, peeled, cored, and diced
- 1/4 cup chopped walnuts
- 1/4 cup maple syrup

INSTRUCTIONS:

1. In a small basin, mix together the eggs, milk, vanilla essence, cinnamon, and salt.
2. In a large pan, melt the butter over medium heat.
3. Dip each piece of bread in the egg mixture, covering both sides equally.

4. Add the bread to the pan and cook for 2-3 minutes each side, or until golden brown.

5. In a small bowl, mix the apples and walnuts.

6. Sprinkle the apple-walnut mixture over the French toast.

7. Drizzle with maple syrup and serve immediately.

Tip:

- For a more luxurious breakfast, top with whipped cream and a sprinkling of cinnamon.

Serving Suggestion: Serve with a side of fruit or yogurt for a full breakfast.

profile image

With the same approach, write for the following diabetic breakfast recipes

TOAST WITH CREAMY AVOCADO AND SPROUTS

- **Prep Time: 5 minutes**
- **Serving Time: 2 minutes**
- **Cooking Time: 0 minutes**

NUTRITIONAL VALUE (PER SERVING):

- Calories: 300
- Fat: 15g
- Saturated Fat: 3g
- Carbohydrates: 30g
- Fiber: 5g
- Sugar: 1g
- Protein: 7g

INGREDIENTS:

- 1-piece whole-wheat bread
- ½ avocado, mashed
- ¼ cup alfalfa sprouts
- A sprinkling of salt and pepper to taste

INSTRUCTIONS:

1. Toast the bread.
2. Spread avocado on the bread.
3. Top with alfalfa sprouts.
4. Season with salt and pepper to taste.
5. Serve immediately.

Tip:

- For more savory toast, add a dab of olive oil or balsamic vinegar.

SCRAMBLED TURMERIC TOFU

- **Prep Time: 10 minutes**
- **Serving Time: 2 minutes**
- **Cooking Time: 10 minutes**

NUTRITIONAL VALUE (PER SERVING):

- Calories: 350
- Fat: 15g

- Saturated Fat: 3g

- Carbohydrates: 30g

- Fiber: 5g

- Sugar: 2g

- Protein: 15g

INGREDIENTS:

- 1 (14-ounce) block firm tofu, drained and crumbled

- 1 tablespoon olive oil

- 1 onion, chopped

- 1 clove garlic, minced

- 1 teaspoon turmeric powder

- ½ teaspoon black pepper

- A pinch of salt

- 2 teaspoons chopped fresh cilantro

INSTRUCTIONS:

1. Heat the olive oil in a large pan over medium heat.

2. Add the onion and garlic and simmer until softened, approximately 5 minutes.

3. Add the tofu, turmeric powder, black pepper, and salt.

4. Cook for 5 minutes, stirring periodically, until the tofu is cooked through.

5. Stir in the cilantro and serve immediately.

Tip:

- For more savory meal, add your favorite veggies, such as broccoli, spinach, or mushrooms.

BREAKFAST SALAD

- **Prep Time: 15 minutes**

- **Serving Time: 2 minutes**

- **Cooking Time: 0 minutes**

NUTRITIONAL VALUE (PER SERVING):

- Calories: 300

- Fat: 10g

- Saturated Fat: 2g

- Carbohydrates: 35g

- Fiber: 5g

- Sugar: 5g

- Protein: 10g

INGREDIENTS:

- 1 cup mixed greens

- ½ cup chopped cooked chicken or tofu

- ¼ cup chopped tomatoes

- ¼ cup chopped cucumber

- 1 tablespoon chopped red onion

- 1 tablespoon olive oil

- 1 tablespoon lemon juice

- A teaspoon of salt and pepper to taste

INSTRUCTIONS:

1. In a large bowl, mix the greens, chicken, tomatoes, cucumber, and red onion.

2. In a small bowl, mix together the olive oil, lemon juice, salt, and pepper.

3. Drizzle the dressing over the salad and toss to coat.

4. Serve immediately.

Tip:

- For more savory salad, add your favorite toppings, such as avocado, nuts, or cheese.

QUINOA BURRITO

- Prep Time: 15 minutes
- Serving Time: 2 minutes
- Cooking Time: 15 minutes

NUTRITIONAL VALUE (PER SERVING):

- Calories: 400
- Fat: 15g
- Saturated Fat: 5g
- Carbohydrates: 50g
- Fiber: 5g
- Sugar: 3g
- Protein: 10g

INGREDIENTS:

- 1 cup cooked quinoa
- 1 (10-inch) whole-wheat tortilla
- ¼ cup refried beans
- ¼ cup chopped cooked chicken or tofu
- ¼ cup chopped tomatoes
- ¼ cup chopped cucumber
- 1 tablespoon chopped red onion
- 1 tablespoon shredded cheese (optional)

INSTRUCTIONS:

1. Warm the tortilla in a dry skillet or microwave for a few seconds.

2. Spread the refried beans on the tortilla.

3. Top with quinoa, chicken, tomatoes, cucumber, red onion, and cheese (if using).

4. Roll up the tortilla securely and serve immediately.

Tip:

- For more savory burrito, add your favorite toppings, such as salsa, sour cream, or guacamole.

BAKED BANANA NUT OATMEAL CUPS

- Prep Time: 15 minutes
- Serving Time: 2 minutes
- Cooking Time: 20 minutes

NUTRITIONAL VALUE (PER SERVING):

- Calories: 350
- Fat: 15g
- Saturated Fat: 3g
- Carbohydrates: 40g
- Fiber: 5g
- Sugar: 10g
- Protein: 7g

INGREDIENTS:

- 1 cup rolled oats
- 1 cup milk
- ½ cup mashed banana
- ¼ cup chopped walnuts
- 2 tablespoons honey
- 1 teaspoon vanilla extract
- ½ teaspoon ground cinnamon
- A pinch of salt

INSTRUCTIONS:

1. Preheat oven to 350 degrees F (175 degrees C).
2. Grease a muffin tray with cooking spray.
3. In a large bowl, mix the oats, milk, banana, walnuts, honey, vanilla essence, cinnamon, and salt.
4. Spoon the mixture into the prepared muffin tray.
5. Bake for 20 minutes, or until golden brown.
6. Let cool slightly before serving.

Tip:

- For more savory dessert, top with fresh fruit or whipped cream.

VEGGIE BREAKFAST WRAP

- **Prep Time: 5 minutes**
- **Serving Time: 2 minutes**
- **Cooking Time: 5 minutes**

NUTRITIONAL VALUE (PER SERVING):

- Calories: 300
- Fat: 10g
- Saturated Fat: 2g
- Carbohydrates: 40g
- Fiber: 5g
- Sugar: 3g
- Protein: 10g

INGREDIENTS:

- 1 (10-inch) whole-wheat tortilla
- 2 scrambled eggs
- ¼ cup chopped spinach
- ¼ cup chopped mushrooms
- ¼ cup chopped tomatoes
- 1 tablespoon shredded cheese (optional)

INSTRUCTIONS:

1. Warm the tortilla in a dry skillet or microwave for a few seconds.

2. Spread the scrambled eggs on the tortilla.

3. Top with spinach, mushrooms, tomatoes, and cheese (if using).

4. Roll up the tortilla securely and serve immediately.

Tip:

- For more savory wrap, add your favorite toppings, such as salsa, sour cream, or guacamole.

BREAKFAST EGG AND HAM BURRITO

- **Prep Time: 5 minutes**
- **Serving Time: 2 minutes**
- **Cooking Time: 10 minutes**

NUTRITIONAL VALUE (PER SERVING):

- Calories: 400
- Fat: 20g
- Saturated Fat: 5g
- Carbohydrates: 30g
- Fiber: 3g
- Sugar: 2g
- Protein: 15g

INGREDIENTS:

- 1 (10-inch) whole-wheat tortilla
- 2 scrambled eggs
- 2 slices cooked ham
- ¼ cup shredded cheese

INSTRUCTIONS:

1. Warm the tortilla in a dry skillet or microwave for a few seconds.

2. Spread the scrambled eggs on the tortilla.

3. Top with ham and cheese.

4. Roll up the tortilla securely and serve immediately.

Tip:

- For more savory tortilla, add your favorite toppings, such as salsa, sour cream, or guacamole

BREAKFAST CUPS FOR MEAT LOVERS

- **Prep Time: 15 minutes**
- **Serving Time: 2 minutes**
- **Cooking Time: 30 minutes**

NUTRITIONAL VALUE (PER SERVING):

- Calories: 450
- Fat: 25g
- Saturated Fat: 10g
- Carbohydrates: 30g
- Fiber: 3g
- Sugar: 2g

Protein: 20g

INGREDIENTS:

- 1 (12-count) muffin tin
- 1 tablespoon olive oil
- 1 onion, chopped
- 1 green bell pepper, chopped
- 1 red bell pepper, chopped
- 1 (15-ounce) can chopped tomatoes, undrained
- 1 teaspoon dried oregano
- ½ teaspoon salt
- ¼ teaspoon black pepper
- 4 big eggs
- 8 slices cooked bacon, crumbled
- 1 cup shredded cheese

INSTRUCTIONS:

1. Preheat oven to 350 degrees F (175 degrees C).
2. Grease the muffin tray with cooking spray.
3. In a large skillet, heat the olive oil over medium heat.
4. Add the onion, bell peppers, and sauté until softened, approximately 5 minutes.
5. Drain the chopped tomatoes, keeping the liquid.
6. Add the diced tomatoes, oregano, salt, and pepper to the skillet.
7. Cook for 5 minutes, stirring periodically.
8. Spoon a dollop of the tomato mixture into each muffin cup.
9. Top with a tablespoon of crumbled bacon.
10. Crack one egg into each muffin cup.
11. Sprinkle with cheese.
12. Bake for 20-25 minutes, or until the eggs are set and the cheese has melted.
13. Let cool slightly before serving.

Tip:

- For more savory breakfast, add your favorite toppings, such as salsa, sour cream, or guacamole.

SUMMER SMOOTHIE FRUIT

- **Prep Time: 5 minutes**
- **Serving Time: 1 minute**
- **Cooking Time: 0 minutes**

NUTRITIONAL VALUE (PER SERVING):

- Calories: 250
- Fat: 5g
- Saturated Fat: 1g
- Carbohydrates: 40g
- Fiber: 5g
- Sugar: 20g
- Protein: 5g

INGREDIENTS:

- 1 cup mixed berries
- 1 cup unsweetened almond milk
- ½ cup frozen mango chunks
- 1 tablespoon honey
- 1 teaspoon ground cinnamon

INSTRUCTIONS:

1. Combine all ingredients in a blender and mix until smooth.
2. Serve immediately.

Tip:

- For a thicker smoothie, add extra almond milk or yogurt. For a thinner smoothie, add extra water or ice.

CHICKEN AND EGG SALAD

- Prep Time: 10 minutes
- Serving Time: 2 minutes
- Cooking Time: 10 minutes

NUTRITIONAL VALUE (PER SERVING):

- Calories: 350
- Fat: 15g
- Saturated Fat: 3g
- Carbohydrates: 20g
- Fiber: 2g
- Sugar: 2g
- Protein: 20g

INGREDIENTS:

- 1 cup cooked chicken, shredded
- 2 hard-boiled eggs, chopped
- ¼ cup chopped celery
- ¼ cup chopped red onion
- 2 tablespoons mayonnaise
- 1 tablespoon lemon juice
- A teaspoon of salt and pepper to taste

INSTRUCTIONS:

1. In a medium bowl, mix the chicken, eggs, celery, red onion, mayonnaise, lemon juice, salt, and pepper.
2. Mix thoroughly and serve immediately.

Tip:

- For tastier salad, add your favorite herbs or spices.

ROLLS WITH SPINACH

- Prep Time: 15 minutes
- Serving Time: 2 minutes
- Cooking Time: 10 minutes

NUTRITIONAL VALUE (PER SERVING):

- Calories: 300
- Fat: 10g
- Saturated Fat: 2g
- Carbohydrates: 40g

- Fiber: 5g
- Sugar: 3g
- Protein: 10g

INGREDIENTS:

- 1 (10x15-inch) sheet puff pastry, thawed if frozen
- 1 cup frozen chopped spinach, thawed and thoroughly drained
- 1 tablespoon olive oil
- ½ cup chopped red onion
- 1 clove garlic, minced
- 1 teaspoon ground cumin
- ½ teaspoon chili powder
- ¼ teaspoon salt
- ¼ teaspoon black pepper
- 1 tablespoon lime juice

INSTRUCTIONS:

1. Preheat oven to 400 degrees F (200 degrees C).
2. To create the filling, heat the olive oil in a large pan over medium heat.
3. Add the onion and garlic and simmer until softened, approximately 5 minutes.
4. Stir in the spinach, cumin, chili powder, salt, and pepper.
5. Cook until the spinach is cooked through, approximately 5 minutes.
6. Stir in the lime juice.
7. Unroll the puff pastry and cut it into 12 rectangles.
8. Place a tablespoon of the spinach filling on each rectangle.
9. Roll up the rectangles and seal the edges.
10. Place the rolls on a baking sheet lined with parchment paper.
11. Bake for 15-20 minutes, or until golden brown.
12. Serve immediately.

Tip:

- For a deeper taste, use mashed avocado instead of diced avocado.

KETO SALAD

- **Prep Time: 10 minutes**
- **Serving Time: 2 minutes**
- **Cooking Time: 0 minutes**

NUTRITIONAL VALUE (PER SERVING):

- Calories: 250
- Fat: 20g
- Saturated Fat: 5g
- Carbohydrates: 5g
- Fiber: 3g
- Sugar: 1g
- Protein: 10g

INGREDIENTS:

- 2 cups mixed greens

- ½ cup chopped avocado
- ¼ cup chopped cucumber
- ¼ cup chopped tomatoes
- ¼ cup chopped red onion
- 2 tablespoons olive oil
- 1 tablespoon lemon juice
- A teaspoon of salt and pepper to taste

INSTRUCTIONS:

1. In a large bowl, mix the greens, avocado, cucumber, tomatoes, and red onion.
2. In a small bowl, mix together the olive oil, lemon juice, salt, and pepper.
3. Drizzle the dressing over the salad and toss to coat.
4. Serve immediately.

Tip:

- For more savory salad, add your favorite toppings, such as nuts, cheese, or grilled chicken.

INSTANT POT CHICKEN CHILI

- **Prep Time: 15 minutes**
- **Cooking Time: 30 minutes**

NUTRITIONAL VALUE (PER SERVING):

- Calories: 400
- Fat: 15g
- Saturated Fat: 5g
- Carbohydrates: 30g
- Fiber: 5g
- Sugar: 2g
- Protein: 20g

INGREDIENTS:

- 1-pound ground chicken
- 1 onion, chopped
- 1 green bell pepper, chopped
- 1 (15-ounce) can chopped tomatoes, undrained
- 1 (15-ounce) can kidney beans, drained and rinsed
- 1 (15-ounce) can black beans, drained and rinsed
- 1 cup beef broth
- 1 tablespoon chili powder
- 1 teaspoon ground cumin
- ½ teaspoon salt
- ¼ teaspoon black pepper
- 1 tablespoon chopped fresh cilantro

INSTRUCTIONS:

1. Set the Instant Pot to sauté mode.
2. Add the ground chicken and heat until browned, approximately 5 minutes.
3. Drain off any excess oil.
4. Add the onion, bell pepper, chopped tomatoes, kidney beans, black beans, beef broth, chili powder, cumin, salt, and pepper.
5. Close the lid and set the valve to sealing.

6. Set the Instant Pot to high pressure and cook for 15 minutes.

7. Let the pressure dissipate naturally for 10 minutes, then remove any leftover pressure manually.

8. Stir in the cilantro and serve immediately.

Tip:

- For a more delicious chili, add diced jalapeño pepper, green onion, or avocado. You may also top with sour cream, cheese, or tortilla chips.

SMOKED CHEESE WRAPS WITH SALMON AND CREAM

- **Prep Time: 10 minutes**
- **Serving Time: 2 minutes**
- **Cooking Time: 0 minutes**

NUTRITIONAL VALUE (PER SERVING):

- Calories: 350
- Fat: 20g
- Saturated Fat: 5g
- Carbohydrates: 25g
- Fiber: 2g
- Sugar: 2g
- Protein: 15g

INGREDIENTS:

- 1 (10-inch) whole-wheat tortilla
- 2 tablespoons cream cheese, softened
- 2 ounces smoked salmon, sliced
- ¼ cup chopped cucumber
- 2 tablespoons chopped red onion
- A teaspoon of salt and pepper to taste

INSTRUCTIONS:

1. Warm the tortilla in a dry skillet or microwave for a few seconds.

2. Spread the cream cheese on the tortilla.

3. Top with smoked salmon, cucumber, red onion, salt, and pepper.

4. Roll up the tortilla securely and serve immediately.

Tip:

- For a more savory wrap, add your favorite toppings, such as capers, dill, or lemon juice.

CHICKEN CHILI

- Prep Time: 15 minutes
- Serving Time: 2 minutes
- Cooking Time: 30 minutes

NUTRITIONAL VALUE (PER SERVING):

- Calories: 350
- Fat: 15g
- Saturated Fat: 5g
- Carbohydrates: 25g
- Fiber: 5g
- Sugar: 2g
- Protein: 20g

INGREDIENTS:

- 1 tablespoon olive oil
- 1 onion, chopped
- 1 green bell pepper, chopped
- 2 cloves garlic, minced
- 1 teaspoon chili powder
- ½ teaspoon ground cumin
- ¼ teaspoon smoked paprika
- A teaspoon of salt and pepper to taste
- 2 cups cooked chicken, shredded
- 1 (15-ounce) can chopped tomatoes, undrained
- 1 (15-ounce) can kidney beans, drained and rinsed
- 1 cup chicken broth

INSTRUCTIONS:

1. Heat the olive oil in a big saucepan over medium heat.
2. Add the onion, bell pepper, and garlic and sauté until softened, approximately 5 minutes.
3. Stir in the chili powder, cumin, paprika, salt, and pepper.
4. Cook for 1 minute longer, stirring regularly.
5. Add the chicken, chopped tomatoes, kidney beans, and chicken broth.
6. Bring to a boil, then decrease heat and simmer for 20 minutes, or until the chili has thickened.
7. Serve immediately.

Tip:

- For a more delicious chili, add diced jalapeño pepper, green onion, or avocado. You may also top with sour cream, cheese, or tortilla chips.

CHICKEN VERA CRUZ

- Prep Time: 15 minutes
- Serving Time: 2 minutes
- Cooking Time: 20 minutes

NUTRITIONAL VALUE (PER SERVING):

- Calories: 300
- Fat: 10g
- Saturated Fat: 2g
- Carbohydrates: 25g
- Fiber: 4g
- Sugar: 3g
- Protein: 20g

INGREDIENTS:

- 1 pound boneless, skinless chicken breasts, cut into bite-sized pieces
- 1 tablespoon olive oil
- 1 onion, chopped
- 1 green bell pepper, chopped
- 1 red bell pepper, chopped
- 1 tomato, chopped
- 1 (15-ounce) can black olives, drained and rinsed
- 1 tablespoon olive oil
- ½ cup chicken broth
- A teaspoon of salt and pepper to taste

INSTRUCTIONS:

1. Heat the olive oil in a large pan over medium heat.
2. Add the chicken and heat until browned on both sides, approximately 5 minutes.
3. Remove the chicken from the skillet and put aside.
4. Add the onion, bell peppers, and tomato to the pan and heat until softened, approximately 5 minutes.
5. Stir in the olives, chicken broth, salt, and pepper.
6. Bring to a boil, then decrease heat and simmer for 5 minutes longer.
7. Return the chicken to the skillet and cook until cooked through, approximately 2 minutes.
8. Serve immediately.

Tip:

- For more savory meal, serve over rice or quinoa.

CHICKEN AND CORNMEAL DUMPLINGS

- **Prep Time: 20 minutes**
- **Serving Time: 2 minutes**
- **Cooking Time: 30 minutes**

NUTRITIONAL VALUE (PER SERVING):

- Calories: 350
- Fat: 15g
- Saturated Fat: 3g
- Carbohydrates: 30g
- Fiber: 4g
- Sugar: 2g
- Protein: 20g

INGREDIENTS:

- 1 pound boneless, skinless chicken breasts, cooked and shredded
- 1 cup boiled chicken broth
- 1 cup cornmeal
- 1 egg
- ¼ cup chopped onion
- ¼ cup chopped celery
- ¼ teaspoon salt
- ¼ teaspoon black pepper

INSTRUCTIONS:

1. In a large bowl, mix the chicken, chicken broth, cornmeal, egg, onion, celery, salt, and pepper.
2. Mix vigorously until a dough forms.
3. Drop by teaspoons into a saucepan of boiling water.
4. Reduce heat and simmer for 15 minutes, or until the dumplings are cooked through.
5. Remove with a slotted spoon and serve immediately.

Tip:

- For more savory meal, add your favorite veggies, such as carrots, peas, or potatoes, to the dough. You may also serve with gravy or your favorite dipping sauce.

CHICKEN AND PEPPERONI

- Prep Time: 10 minutes
- Serving Time: 2 minutes
- Cooking Time: 20 minutes

NUTRITIONAL VALUE (PER SERVING):

- Calories: 300
- Fat: 15g
- Saturated Fat: 5g
- Carbohydrates: 15g
- Fiber: 2g
- Sugar: 2g
- Protein: 25g

INGREDIENTS:

- 1 pound boneless, skinless chicken breasts, cut into bite-sized pieces
- 1 tablespoon olive oil
- 1 onion, chopped
- 1 green bell pepper, chopped
- ½ cup sliced pepperoni
- ½ cup shredded mozzarella cheese
- A teaspoon of salt and pepper to taste

INSTRUCTIONS:

1. Heat the olive oil in a large pan over medium heat.
2. Add the chicken and heat until browned on both sides, approximately 5 minutes.

3. Add the onion, bell pepper, and pepperoni and simmer until the veggies are cooked, approximately 5 minutes longer.

4. Stir in the mozzarella cheese and simmer until melted.

5. Season with salt and pepper to taste.

6. Serve immediately.

Tip:

- For more savory meal, add your preferred herbs or spices, such as oregano, garlic powder, or red pepper flakes. You may also serve over spaghetti for a full dinner.

CHICKEN AND SAUSAGE GUMBO

- **Prep Time: 30 minutes**
- **Serving Time: 5 minutes**
- **Cooking Time: 1 hour**

NUTRITIONAL VALUE (PER SERVING):

- Calories: 450
- Fat: 20g
- Saturated Fat: 5g
- Carbohydrates: 30g
- Fiber: 5g
- Sugar: 2g
- Protein: 30g

INGREDIENTS:

- 1 tablespoon olive oil
- 1 onion, chopped
- 1 green bell pepper, chopped
- 1 red bell pepper, chopped
- 2 cloves garlic, minced
- 1 teaspoon chili powder
- ½ teaspoon ground cumin
- ¼ teaspoon cayenne pepper
- A teaspoon of salt and pepper to taste
- 1 pound boneless, skinless chicken breasts, cut into bite-sized pieces
- 1 pound smoked sausage, sliced
- 1 (15-ounce) can chopped tomatoes, undrained
- 1 (15-ounce) can chicken broth
- 1 cup cooked white rice

INSTRUCTIONS:

1. Heat the olive oil in a big saucepan over medium heat.

2. Add the onion, bell peppers, and garlic and sauté until softened, approximately 5 minutes.

3. Stir in the chili powder, cumin, cayenne pepper, salt, and pepper.

4. Cook for 1 minute longer, stirring regularly.

5. Add the chicken, sausage, chopped tomatoes, and chicken broth.

6. Bring to a boil, then decrease heat and simmer for 45 minutes, or until the chicken is cooked through.

7. Stir in the rice and simmer for 5 minutes longer, or until the rice is cooked through.

8. Serve immediately.

Tip:

- For a more delicious gumbo, add chopped jalapeño pepper, green onion, or avocado. You may also top with sour cream, cheese, or tortilla chips.

CHICKEN, BARLEY, AND LEEK STEW

- **Prep Time: 15 minutes**
- **Serving Time: 2 minutes**
- **Cooking Time: 30 minutes**

NUTRITIONAL VALUE (PER SERVING):

- Calories: 350
- Fat: 10g
- Saturated Fat: 2g
- Carbohydrates: 35g
- Fiber: 5g
- Sugar: 3g
- Protein: 20g

INGREDIENTS:

- 1 tablespoon olive oil
- 2 leeks, white and light green portions only, thinly sliced
- 2 cloves garlic, minced
- 2 cups cooked chicken, shredded
- 1 cup boiled barley
- 4 cups chicken broth
- A teaspoon of salt and pepper to taste

INSTRUCTIONS:

1. Heat the olive oil in a big saucepan over medium heat.

2. Add the leeks and simmer until softened, approximately 5 minutes.

3. Stir in the garlic and simmer for 1 minute longer, stirring frequently.

4. Add the chicken, barley, chicken broth, salt, and pepper.

5. Bring to a boil, then decrease heat and simmer for 15 minutes, or until the barley is soft.

6. Serve immediately.

Tip:

- For more savory stew, add your favorite veggies, such as carrots, celery, or potatoes, to the pot. You may also serve with a dollop of sour cream or a sprinkling of fresh herbs.

CIDER PORK STEW

- **Prep Time: 20 minutes**
- **Serving Time: 2 minutes**
- **Cooking Time: 1 hour**

NUTRITIONAL VALUE (PER SERVING):

- Calories: 400
- Fat: 20g
- Saturated Fat: 5g
- Carbohydrates: 30g
- Fiber: 4g
- Sugar: 5g
- Protein: 25g

INGREDIENTS:

- 2 tablespoons olive oil
- 2 onions, chopped
- 2 carrots, chopped
- 2 celery stalks, chopped
- 2 cloves garlic, minced
- 1 teaspoon ground cumin
- ½ teaspoon ground coriander
- ¼ teaspoon ground cinnamon
- A teaspoon of salt and pepper to taste
- 2 pounds boneless, skinless pork shoulder, sliced into bite-sized pieces
- 1 (28-ounce) can apple cider
- 1 cup beef broth

INSTRUCTIONS:

1. Heat the olive oil in a big saucepan over medium heat.
2. Add the onion, carrots, celery, and garlic and simmer until softened, approximately 10 minutes
3. Stir in the cumin, coriander, cinnamon, salt, and pepper.
4. Cook for 1 minute longer, stirring regularly.
5. Add the pork and heat until browned on both sides, approximately 5 minutes.
6. Stir in the apple cider and beef broth.
7. Bring to a boil, then decrease heat and simmer for 1 hour, or until the pork is cooked.
8. Serve immediately.

Tip:

- For a more delicious stew, add chopped apples or pears to the pot. You may also serve with a dollop of sour cream or a sprinkling of fresh herbs.

CREAMY CHICKEN NOODLE SOUP

- **Prep Time: 15 minutes**
- **Serving Time: 2 minutes**
- **Cooking Time: 30 minutes**

- Calories: 350
- Fat: 15g
- Saturated Fat: 5g
- Carbohydrates: 25g
- Fiber: 3g
- Sugar: 2g
- Protein: 20g

INGREDIENTS:

- 2 tablespoons butter
- 1 onion, chopped
- 2 carrots, chopped
- 2 celery stalks, chopped
- 2 cloves garlic, minced
- 1 teaspoon dried thyme
- ¼ teaspoon salt
- ¼ teaspoon black pepper
- 4 cups chicken broth
- 1 cup cooked chicken, shredded
- ½ cup thick cream
- 2 cups broad egg noodles

INSTRUCTIONS:

1. In a large saucepan, melt the butter over medium heat.
2. Add the onion, carrots, celery, and garlic and simmer until softened, approximately 5 minutes.
3. Stir in the thyme, salt, and pepper.
4. Cook for 1 minute longer, stirring regularly.
5. Add the chicken broth and bring to a boil.
6. Reduce heat and simmer for 10 minutes.
7. Stir in the chicken, heavy cream, and egg noodles.
8. Cook for 5 minutes longer, or until the noodles are soft.
9. Serve immediately.

Tip:

- For a more delicious soup, add chopped vegetables, such as peas, corn, or green beans, to the pot. You may also top with grated Parmesan cheese or a dab of sour cream.

GAZPACHO

- Prep Time: 15 minutes
- Serving Time: 2 minutes
- Cooking Time: 0 minutes

NUTRITIONAL VALUE (PER SERVING):

- Calories: 200
- Fat: 5g
- Saturated Fat: 1g
- Carbohydrates: 20g
- Fiber: 3g

- Sugar: 10g
- Protein: 3g

INGREDIENTS:

- 2 pounds' ripe tomatoes, cored and seeded
- 1 cucumber, peeled and seeded
- 1 green bell pepper, cored and seeded
- 1 onion, chopped
- 2 cloves garlic, minced
- 1 tablespoon olive oil
- 1 tablespoon red wine vinegar
- A teaspoon of salt and pepper to taste

INSTRUCTIONS:

1. In a blender, add the tomatoes, cucumber, bell pepper, onion, garlic, olive oil, vinegar, salt, and pepper.
2. Blend until smooth.
3. Chill in the refrigerator for at least 2 hours before serving.

Tip:

- For more savory gazpacho, add your favorite herbs, such as cilantro, basil, or oregano. You may also top with chopped veggies, such as tomatoes, cucumbers, or bell peppers.

TOMATO AND KALE SOUP

- Prep Time: 15 minutes
- Serving Time: 2 minutes
- Cooking Time: 30 minutes

NUTRITIONAL VALUE (PER SERVING):

- Calories: 250
- Fat: 5g
- Saturated Fat: 1g
- Carbohydrates: 25g
- Fiber: 4g
- Sugar: 5g
- Protein: 5g

INGREDIENTS:

- 2 tablespoons olive oil
- 1 onion, chopped
- 2 cloves garlic, minced
- 1 (28-ounce) can crushed tomatoes
- 1 (15-ounce) can chopped tomatoes, undrained
- 4 cups chicken broth
- 1 bunch kale, stems and cut
- A teaspoon of salt and pepper to taste

INSTRUCTIONS:

1. Heat the olive oil in a big saucepan over medium heat.
2. Add the onion and simmer until softened, approximately 5 minutes.
3. Stir in the garlic and simmer for 1 minute longer, stirring frequently.

4. Add the crushed tomatoes, diced tomatoes, chicken stock, kale, salt, and pepper.

5. Bring to a boil, then decrease heat and simmer for 20 minutes, or until the kale is soft.

6. Serve immediately.

Tip:

- For more savory soup, add your favorite herbs, such as oregano, basil, or rosemary. You may also top with grated Parmesan cheese or a dab of sour cream.

COMFORTING SUMMER SQUASH SOUP WITH CRISPY CHICKPEAS

- Prep Time: 20 minutes
- Serving Time: 2 minutes
- Cooking Time: 30 minutes

NUTRITIONAL VALUE (PER SERVING):

- Calories: 300
- Fat: 10g
- Saturated Fat: 2g
- Carbohydrates: 35g
- Fiber: 5g
- Sugar: 5g
- Protein: 10g

INGREDIENTS:

- 2 tablespoons olive oil
- 1 onion, chopped
- 2 cloves garlic, minced
- 2 pounds' yellow summer squash, halved and seeded
- 1 cup chicken broth
- A teaspoon of salt and pepper to taste

For the Crispy Chickpeas:

- 1 (15-ounce) can chickpeas, drained and rinsed
- 1 tablespoon olive oil
- ½ teaspoon cumin
- ¼ teaspoon chili powder
- A teaspoon of salt and pepper to taste

INSTRUCTIONS:

1. Heat the olive oil in a big saucepan over medium heat.

2. Add the onion and simmer until softened, approximately 5 minutes.

3. Stir in the garlic and simmer for 1 minute longer, stirring frequently.

4. Add the summer squash and chicken broth.

5. Bring to a boil, then decrease heat and simmer for 20 minutes, or until the squash is soft.

6. Use an immersion blender or normal blender to purée the soup until smooth.

7. Season with salt and pepper to taste.

To make the crispy chickpeas:

1. Preheat oven to 400 degrees F (200 degrees C).
2. In a medium bowl, stir the chickpeas with the olive oil, cumin, chili powder, salt, and pepper.
3. Spread the chickpeas on a baking sheet in a single layer.
4. Bake for 20 minutes, or until the chickpeas are crispy.

To serve:

1. Ladle the soup into bowls.
2. Top with crispy chickpeas.
3. Serve immediately.

Tip:

- For more savory soup, add your favorite herbs, such as basil, oregano, or parsley. You may also top with a dollop of sour cream or a sprinkle of olive oil.

CURRIED CARROT SOUP

- Prep Time: 15 minutes
- Serving Time: 2 minutes
- Cooking Time: 30 minutes

NUTRITIONAL VALUE (PER SERVING):

- Calories: 250
- Fat: 5g
- Saturated Fat: 1g
- Carbohydrates: 25g
- Fiber: 4g
- Sugar: 5g
- Protein: 5g

INGREDIENTS:

- 2 tablespoons olive oil
- 1 onion, chopped
- 2 cloves garlic, minced
- 2 pounds' carrots, peeled and sliced
- 1 tablespoon curry powder
- 1 teaspoon ground ginger
- ¼ teaspoon cayenne pepper
- 4 cups chicken broth
- A teaspoon of salt and pepper to taste

INSTRUCTIONS:

1. Heat the olive oil in a big saucepan over medium heat.
2. Add the onion and simmer until softened, approximately 5 minutes.
3. Stir in the garlic and simmer for 1 minute longer, stirring frequently.
4. Add the carrots, curry powder, ginger, and cayenne pepper.
5. Cook for 5 minutes, stirring regularly, to roast the spices.
6. Add the chicken broth.

7. Bring to a boil, then decrease heat and simmer for 20 minutes, or until the carrots are soft.

8. Use an immersion blender or normal blender to purée the soup until smooth.

9. Season with salt and pepper to taste.

Tip:

- For more savory soup, add your favorite herbs, such as cilantro, parsley, or mint. You may also top with a dollop of sour cream or a sprinkling of toasted nuts.

THAI PEANUT, CARROT, AND SHRIMP SOUP

- **Prep Time: 15 minutes**
- **Serving Time: 2 minutes**
- **Cooking Time: 20 minutes**

NUTRITIONAL VALUE (PER SERVING):

- Calories: 350
- Fat: 15g
- Saturated Fat: 5g
- Carbohydrates: 25g
- Fiber: 3g
- Sugar: 2g
- Protein: 20g

INGREDIENTS:

- 1 tablespoon olive oil
- 1 onion, chopped
- 2 cloves garlic, minced
- 1 pound carrots, peeled and sliced
- 1 (14-ounce) can light coconut milk
- 2 tbsp. peanut butter
- 2 teaspoons fish sauce
- 1 tablespoon lime juice
- A pinch of red pepper flakes
- 1-pound shrimp, peeled and deveined
- A teaspoon of salt and pepper to taste

INSTRUCTIONS:

1. Heat the olive oil in a big saucepan over medium heat.

2. Add the onion and simmer until softened, approximately 5 minutes.

3. Stir in the garlic and simmer for 1 minute longer, stirring frequently.

4. Add the carrots, coconut milk, peanut butter, fish sauce, lime juice, and red pepper flakes.

5. Bring to a boil, then decrease heat and simmer for 10 minutes.

6. Add the shrimp and heat until pink and cooked through, approximately 3-5 minutes.

7. Season with salt and pepper to taste.

Tip:

- For more savory soup, add your favorite herbs, such as cilantro, basil, or mint. You may also top with chopped peanuts or a dollop of sour cream.

CHICKEN TORTILLA SOUP

- **Prep Time: 20 minutes**
- **Serving Time: 2 minutes**
- **Cooking Time: 30 minutes**

NUTRITIONAL VALUE (PER SERVING):

- Calories: 400
- Fat: 15g
- Saturated Fat: 5g
- Carbohydrates: 30g
- Fiber: 4g
- Sugar: 2g
- Protein: 25g

INGREDIENTS:

- 2 tablespoons olive oil
- 1 onion, chopped
- 2 cloves garlic, minced
- 1 pound boneless, skinless chicken breasts, cooked and shredded
- 1 (28-ounce) can chopped tomatoes, undrained
- 1 (15-ounce) can black beans, drained and rinsed
- 1 (15-ounce) can corn kernels, drained and rinsed
- 4 cups chicken broth
- 1 teaspoon chili powder
- ½ teaspoon ground cumin
- A teaspoon of salt and pepper to taste
- 8 tortilla chips, for garnish

INSTRUCTIONS:

1. Heat the olive oil in a big saucepan over medium heat.
2. Add the onion and simmer until softened, approximately 5 minutes.
3. Stir in the garlic and simmer for 1 minute longer, stirring frequently.
4. Add the shredded chicken, chopped tomatoes, black beans, corn kernels, chicken broth, chili powder, cumin, salt, and pepper.
5. Bring to a boil, then decrease heat and simmer for 20 minutes, or until the flavors have merged.
6. To serve, spoon the soup into bowls and top with tortilla chips.

Tip:

- For more savory soup, add your favorite toppings, such as chopped cilantro, avocado, sour cream, or grated cheese. You may also add a pinch of cayenne pepper for a touch more flavor.

BEEF AND MUSHROOM BARLEY SOUP

- Prep Time: 15 minutes
- Serving Time: 2 minutes
- Cooking Time: 45 minutes

NUTRITIONAL VALUE (PER SERVING):

- Calories: 400
- Fat: 20g
- Saturated Fat: 5g
- Carbohydrates: 35g
- Fiber: 5g
- Sugar: 2g
- Protein: 25g

INGREDIENTS:

- 2 tablespoons olive oil
- 1 pound boneless, skinless beef chuck, cut into bite-sized pieces
- 1 onion, chopped
- 2 carrots, chopped
- 2 celery stalks, chopped
- 2 cloves garlic, minced
- 1 teaspoon dried thyme
- ½ teaspoon dried rosemary
- A teaspoon of salt and pepper to taste
- 4 cups beef broth
- 1 cup boiled barley
- 8 ounces sliced mushrooms

INSTRUCTIONS:

1. Heat the olive oil in a big saucepan over medium heat.
2. Add the steak and heat until browned on both sides, approximately 5 minutes.
3. Remove the steak from the saucepan and put aside.
4. Add the onion, carrots, celery, and garlic to the saucepan and simmer until softened, approximately 5 minutes.
5. Stir in the thyme, rosemary, salt, and pepper.
6. Cook for 1 minute longer, stirring regularly.
7. Return the meat to the saucepan and whisk in the beef broth, barley, and mushrooms.
8. Bring to a boil, then decrease heat and simmer for 30 minutes, or until the meat is cooked.
9. Serve immediately.

Tip:

- For more savory soup, add your favorite veggies, such as peas, corn, or green beans, to the pot. You may also top with grated Parmesan cheese or a dab of sour cream.

TOMATO AND GUACA SALAD

- Prep Time: 10 minutes

- Serving Time: 2 minutes
- Cooking Time: 0 minutes

NUTRITIONAL VALUE (PER SERVING):

- Calories: 250
- Fat: 10g
- Saturated Fat: 2g
- Carbohydrates: 25g
- Fiber: 5g
- Sugar: 5g
- Protein: 5g

INGREDIENTS:

- 2 pounds' ripe tomatoes, diced
- 1 avocado, mashed
- 1 tablespoon red onion, chopped
- 1 tablespoon cilantro, chopped
- 1 tablespoon lime juice
- A teaspoon of salt and pepper to taste

INSTRUCTIONS:

1. In a large bowl, mix the tomatoes, avocado, red onion, cilantro, lime juice, salt, and pepper.
2. Toss to coat.
3. Serve immediately.

Tip:

- For a more delicious salad, add your favorite toppings, such as diced cucumbers, jalapenos, or grated cheese. You may also serve with tortilla chips or pita bread.

COLESLAW

- Prep Time: 10 minutes
- Serving Time: 2 minutes
- Cooking Time: 0 minutes

NUTRITIONAL VALUE (PER SERVING):

- Calories: 150
- Fat: 5g
- Saturated Fat: 1g
- Carbohydrates: 15g
- Fiber: 3g
- Sugar: 5g
- Protein: 2g

INGREDIENTS:

- 1 head cabbage, shredded
- 1 carrot, shredded
- ½ cup mayonnaise
- 2 teaspoons apple cider vinegar
- 1 tablespoon Dijon mustard
- 1 tablespoon sugar
- A teaspoon of salt and pepper to taste

INSTRUCTIONS:

1. In a large bowl, mix the cabbage, carrot, mayonnaise, vinegar, mustard, sugar, salt, and pepper.

2. Toss to coat.

3. Serve immediately or refrigerate for later.

Tip:

- For a more delicious coleslaw, add your favorite toppings, such as chopped celery, red onion, or green beans. You may also serve with a sprinkling of paprika or a drizzle of honey.

GREEN SALAD WITH BERRIES AND SWEET POTATOES

- **Prep Time: 15 minutes**
- **Serving Time: 2 minutes**
- **Cooking Time: 10 minutes**

NUTRITIONAL VALUE (PER SERVING):

- Calories: 350
- Fat: 15g
- Saturated Fat: 3g
- Carbohydrates: 30g
- Fiber: 4g
- Sugar: 5g
- Protein: 5g

INGREDIENTS:

- 4 cups mixed greens
- 1 cup roasted sweet potatoes, diced
- ½ cup blueberries
- ¼ cup sliced almonds
- 2 tablespoons olive oil
- 1 tablespoon balsamic vinegar
- A teaspoon of salt and pepper to taste

INSTRUCTIONS:

1. Preheat oven to 400 degrees F (200 degrees C).

2. Toss the sweet potatoes with olive oil, salt, and pepper.

3. Spread the sweet potatoes on a baking sheet and roast for 10 minutes, or until soft.

4. In a large bowl, mix the greens, roasted sweet potatoes, blueberries, and almonds.

5. In a small bowl, mix together the olive oil, balsamic vinegar, salt, and pepper.

6. Drizzle the dressing over the salad and toss to coat.

7. Serve immediately.

Tip:

- For more savory salad, add your favorite toppings, such as diced avocado, feta cheese, or a sprinkling of sunflower seeds. You may also serve with a grilled chicken breast or a salmon fillet.

- **Prep Time: 10 minutes**
- **Serving Time: 2 minutes**
- **Cooking Time: 0 minutes**

NUTRITIONAL VALUE (PER SERVING):

- Calories: 200
- Fat: 5g
- Saturated Fat: 1g
- Carbohydrates: 30g
- Fiber: 3g
- Sugar: 10g
- Protein: 2g

INGREDIENTS:

- 2 cups mixed fruit, such as strawberries, blueberries, raspberries, and grapes
- ¼ cup honey
- 2 teaspoons lime juice
- A pinch of salt

INSTRUCTIONS:

1. In a large dish, add the mixed fruit.
2. In a small bowl, stir together the honey, lime juice, and salt.
3. Drizzle the dressing over the fruit salad and toss to coat.
4. Serve immediately.

Tip:

- For more savory fruit salad, add your favorite toppings, such as diced mango, pineapple, or kiwi. You may also top with a dab of whipped cream or a sprinkling of granola.

CHOCOLATE-COVERED STRAWBERRIES

- **Prep Time: 10 minutes**
- **Serving Time: 2 minutes**
- **Cooking Time: 0 minutes**

NUTRITIONAL VALUE (PER SERVING):

- Calories: 150
- Fat: 10g
- Saturated Fat: 6g
- Carbohydrates: 15g
- Fiber: 2g
- Sugar: 10g
- Protein: 2g

INGREDIENTS:

- 1 pound strawberries, hulled
- 1 (8-ounce) container semisweet chocolate chips, melted

INSTRUCTIONS:

1. Dip each strawberry into the melted chocolate.

2. Place the chocolate-covered strawberries on a baking sheet lined with parchment paper.

3. Refrigerate until the chocolate is set, approximately 15 minutes.

4. Serve immediately.

Tip:

- For more savory treat, add your favorite toppings, such as sprinkles, chopped nuts, or dried fruit. You may also serve with a glass of milk or sparkling water.

BEAN AND SCALLION SALAD

- Prep Time: 10 minutes
- Serving Time: 2 minutes
- Cooking Time: 0 minutes

NUTRITIONAL VALUE (PER SERVING):

- Calories: 250
- Fat: 10g
- Saturated Fat: 2g
- Carbohydrates: 25g
- Fiber: 5g
- Sugar: 5g
- Protein: 5g

INGREDIENTS:

- 1 (15-ounce) can kidney beans, drained and rinsed
- 1 (15-ounce) can black beans, drained and rinsed
- 1 (15-ounce) can garbanzo beans, drained and rinsed
- ¼ cup chopped scallions
- ¼ cup prepared vinaigrette dressing

INSTRUCTIONS:

1. In a large dish, mix the drained and rinsed beans, chopped scallions, and dressing.

2. Toss to coat.

3. Serve immediately.

Tip:

- For more savory salad, add your favorite toppings, such as diced tomatoes, cucumbers, or avocado. You may also top with a dollop of sour cream or a sprinkling of paprika.

RAINBOW BEAN SALAD

- Prep Time: 15 minutes
- Serving Time: 2 minutes
- Cooking Time: 0 minutes

NUTRITIONAL VALUE (PER SERVING):

- Calories: 300

- Fat: 15g
- Saturated Fat: 3g
- Carbohydrates: 30g
- Fiber: 5g
- Sugar: 5g
- Protein: 6g

INGREDIENTS:

- 1 (15-ounce) can kidney beans, drained and rinsed
- 1 (15-ounce) can black beans, drained and rinsed
- 1 (15-ounce) can garbanzo beans, drained and rinsed
- 1 cup chopped red bell peppers
- 1 cup chopped cucumber
- ½ cup chopped corn kernels ¼ cup chopped red onion
- ¼ cup prepared vinaigrette dressing

INSTRUCTIONS:

1. In a large bowl, mix the drained and rinsed beans, chopped veggies, and dressing.
2. Toss to coat.
3. Serve immediately.

Tip:

- For a more vibrant salad, add your favorite veggies, such as diced yellow bell peppers, chopped celery, or black olives. You may also top with a dollop of sour cream or a sprinkling of shredded cheese.

WARM BARLEY AND SQUASH SALAD

- Prep Time: 15 minutes
- Serving Time: 2 minutes
- Cooking Time: 15 minutes

NUTRITIONAL VALUE (PER SERVING):

- Calories: 350
- Fat: 15g
- Saturated Fat: 3g
- Carbohydrates: 35g
- Fiber: 6g
- Sugar: 5g
- Protein: 5g

INGREDIENTS:

- 1 cup boiled barley
- 1 cup chopped butternut squash
- ½ cup chopped red onion
- ¼ cup chopped celery ¼ cup chopped walnuts
- ¼ cup prepared vinaigrette dressing

INSTRUCTIONS:

1. Preheat oven to 400 degrees F (200 degrees C).

2. Toss the chopped butternut squash with olive oil, salt, and pepper.

3. Spread the squash on a baking sheet and roast for 15 minutes, or until soft.

4. In a large bowl, mix the cooked barley, roasted butternut squash, chopped veggies, walnuts, and dressing.

5. Toss to coat.

6. Serve immediately.

Tip:

- For more savory salad, add your favorite toppings, such as dried cranberries, goat cheese, or a drizzle of honey. You may also sprinkle with cinnamon.

CITRUS AND CHICKEN SALAD

- **Prep Time: 20 minutes**
- **Serving Time: 2 minutes**
- **Cooking Time: 0 minutes**

NUTRITIONAL VALUE (PER SERVING):

- Calories: 350
- Fat: 15g
- Saturated Fat: 4g
- Carbohydrates: 25g
- Fiber: 5g
- Sugar: 5g
- Protein: 25g

INGREDIENTS:

- 2 cups cooked chicken, shredded
- ½ cup chopped oranges
- ½ cup diced grapefruit ¼ cup chopped red onion
- ¼ cup prepared vinaigrette dressing

INSTRUCTIONS:

1. In a large bowl, add the cooked chicken, diced oranges, chopped grapefruit, chopped red onion, and dressing.

2. Toss to coat.

3. Serve immediately.

Reciepe Card

COURSE: DIET: PREP TIME: COOK TIME: SERVINGS

INGREDIENTS

INSTRUCTIONS

Serves   Prep   Cook Time

TIPS & TRICKS

NOTES

PORK CHOP DIANE

- Prep Time: 15 minutes
- Serving Time: 2 minutes
- Cooking Time: 10 minutes

NUTRITIONAL VALUE (PER SERVING):

Calories: 350 | Fat: 20g | Saturated Fat: 5g | Carbohydrates: 10g | Fiber: 2g | Sugar: 5g | Protein: 30g

INGREDIENTS:

- 2 boneless, center-cut pork chops (approximately 1-pound total)
- 1 tablespoon olive oil
- Salt and pepper to taste
- 2 tablespoons butter
- 2 teaspoons Worcestershire sauce
- 1/4 cup beef broth
- 1/4 cup dry white wine
- 1 tablespoon Dijon mustard
- 2 teaspoons chopped fresh parsley

INSTRUCTIONS:

1. Pat the pork chops dry with paper towels and season with salt and pepper.
2. Heat the olive oil in a large pan over medium-high heat.
3. Add the pork chops and heat for 3-4 minutes each side, or until browned.
4. Remove the pork chops from the pan and put aside.
5. Add the butter to the pan and melt over medium heat.
6. Stir in the Worcestershire sauce, beef broth, wine, mustard, and parsley.
7. Bring to a boil and cook for 5 minutes, or until the sauce has thickened.
8. Return the pork chops to the pan and coat with the sauce.
9. Serve immediately.

Tip:

- For more savory dinner, serve the pork chops with a side of roasted vegetables, such as carrots, parsnips, or Brussels sprouts.

AUTUMN PORK CHOPS WITH RED CABBAGE AND APPLES

- Prep Time: 20 minutes
- Serving Time: 2 minutes
- Cooking Time: 20 minutes

NUTRITIONAL VALUE (PER SERVING):

Calories: 300 | Fat: 15g | Saturated Fat: 5g | Carbohydrates: 20g | Fiber: 3g | Sugar: 5g | Protein: 25g

INGREDIENTS:

- 2 boneless, center-cut pork chops (approximately 1-pound total)
- 1 tablespoon olive oil
- Salt and pepper to taste
- 1/2 head of red cabbage, thinly sliced
- 1 apple, cored and thinly sliced
- 1/4 cup chicken broth
- 1 tablespoon Dijon mustard
- 1 tablespoon honey
- 1 teaspoon ground cinnamon
- 1/4 teaspoon ground nutmeg

INSTRUCTIONS:

1. Preheat oven to 375 degrees F (190 degrees C).
2. Pat the pork chops dry with paper towels and season with salt and pepper.
3. Heat the olive oil in a large pan over medium-high heat.
4. Add the pork chops and heat for 3-4 minutes each side, or until browned.
5. Remove the pork chops from the pan and put aside.
6. Add the red cabbage and apple to the pan and simmer over medium heat for 5 minutes, or until the cabbage has softened.
7. Stir in the chicken broth, mustard, honey, cinnamon, and nutmeg.
8. Bring to a boil and cook for 5 minutes, or until the sauce has thickened.
9. Place the pork chops on a baking dish and pour the sauce over them.
10. Bake for 15-20 minutes, or until the pork chops are cooked through.
11. Serve immediately.

Tip:

- For more savory meal, add a dollop of sour cream or crème fraîche to the pork chops before serving.

ORANGE-MARINATED PORK TENDERLOIN

- **Prep Time: 15 minutes**
- **Serving Time: 2 hours**
- **Cooking Time: 20 minutes**

NUTRITIONAL VALUE (PER SERVING):

Calories: 250 | Fat: 10g | Saturated Fat: 3g | Carbohydrates: 15g | Fiber: 2g | Sugar: 5g | Protein: 25g

INGREDIENTS:

- 1-pound pork tenderloin, trimmed
- 1/4 cup orange juice
- 1 tablespoon soy sauce
- 1 tablespoon honey
- 1 tablespoon Dijon mustard

- 1 teaspoon grated orange zest
- Salt and pepper to taste

INSTRUCTIONS:

1. In a large bowl, mix together the orange juice, soy sauce, honey, mustard, and orange zest.
2. Add the pork tenderloin to the bowl and toss to coat.
3. Cover and refrigerate for at least 2 hours, or up to overnight.
4. Preheat oven to 400 degrees F (200 degrees C).
5. Remove the pork tenderloin from the marinade and discard the marinade.
6. Place the pork tenderloin in a baking dish and season with salt and pepper.
7. Bake for 20-25 minutes, or until the pork tenderloin is cooked through.
8. Serve immediately.

Tip:

- For more savory dinner, serve the pork tenderloin with a side of roasted vegetables, such as carrots, parsnips, or Brussels sprouts.

CITRUS AND CHICKEN SALAD

- **Prep Time: 20 minutes**
- **Serving Time: 2 minutes**
- **Cooking Time: 0 minutes**

NUTRITIONAL VALUE (PER SERVING):

- Calories: 350
- Fat: 15g
- Saturated Fat: 4g
- Carbohydrates: 25g
- Fiber: 5g
- Sugar: 5g
- Protein: 25g

INGREDIENTS:

- 2 cups cooked chicken, shredded
- ½ cup canned mandarin oranges, drained
- ½ cup chopped grapefruit segments
- ¼ cup chopped red onion
- ¼ cup prepared vinaigrette dressing

INSTRUCTIONS:

1. In a large bowl, add the shredded chicken, canned mandarin oranges, grapefruit segments, chopped red onion, and vinaigrette dressing.
2. Toss to coat.
3. Serve immediately.

Tip:

- For more savory salad, add a dollop of sour cream or crème fraîche to the salad before serving. You may also add a sprinkling of chopped herbs, such as fresh parsley or cilantro.

BLUEBERRY AND CHICKEN SALAD

- Prep Time: 20 minutes
- Serving Time: 2 minutes
- Cooking Time: 0 minutes

NUTRITIONAL VALUE (PER SERVING):

- Calories: 400
- Fat: 20g
- Saturated Fat: 5g
- Carbohydrates: 30g
- Fiber: 5g
- Sugar: 5g
- Protein: 25g

INGREDIENTS:

- 2 cups cooked chicken, shredded
- ½ cup blueberries
- ¼ cup chopped celery
- ¼ cup chopped walnuts
- ¼ cup prepared vinaigrette dressing

INSTRUCTIONS:

1. In a large bowl, add the shredded chicken, blueberries, sliced celery, chopped walnuts, and vinaigrette dressing.
2. Toss to coat.
3. Serve immediately.

Tip:

- For a more delicious salad, add a sprinkle of dried cranberries or diced grapes to the salad before serving. You may also add a sprinkle of honey or maple syrup.

LIME-PARSLEY LAMB CUTLETS

- Prep Time: 10 minutes
- Serving Time: 2 minutes
- Cooking Time: 5 minutes

NUTRITIONAL VALUE (PER SERVING):

- Calories: 300
- Fat: 15g
- Saturated Fat: 5g
- Carbohydrates: 5g
- Fiber: 1g
- Sugar: 2g
- Protein: 30g

INGREDIENTS:

- 4 lamb cutlets (approximately 1-pound total)
- 1 tablespoon olive oil
- Salt and pepper to taste
- 1 tablespoon lime juice
- 1 tablespoon chopped fresh parsley

INSTRUCTIONS:

1. Pat the lamb cutlets dry with paper towels and season with salt and pepper.

2. Heat the olive oil in a large pan over medium-high heat.

3. Add the lamb cutlets and fry for 2-3 minutes each side, or until browned and cooked through.

4. In a small bowl, mix together the lime juice and parsley.

5. Drizzle the lime-parsley sauce over the lamb cutlets.

6. Serve immediately.

Tip:

- For more savory dinner, serve the lamb cutlets with a side of roasted vegetables, such as asparagus, zucchini, or bell peppers.

BEEF FAJITAS

- **Prep Time: 15 minutes**
- **Cooking Time: 10 minutes**
- **Serving Time: 5 minutes**

NUTRITIONAL VALUE (PER SERVING):

- Calories: 400
- Fat: 20g
- Saturated Fat: 7g
- Carbohydrates: 35g
- Fiber: 5g
- Sugar: 5g
- Protein: 30g

INGREDIENTS:

- 1-pound flank steak, thinly sliced
- 1 tablespoon olive oil
- 1 onion, thinly sliced
- 1 green bell pepper, finely sliced
- 1 red bell pepper, thinly sliced
- 1 tablespoon chili powder
- 1 teaspoon ground cumin
- 1/2 teaspoon salt
- 1/4 teaspoon black pepper

INSTRUCTIONS:

1. In a large bowl, mix the sliced flank steak, olive oil, onion, green bell pepper, red bell pepper, chili powder, cumin, salt, and pepper.

2. Toss to coat.

3. Heat a large skillet over medium-high heat.

4. Add the meat mixture and heat for 5-7 minutes, or until the steak is cooked through and the veggies are soft.

5. Serve immediately with warm tortillas, your favorite toppings, such as shredded cheese, sour cream, guacamole, and salsa.

Tips:

- For a more delicious marinade, marinate the sliced beef in the mixture for at least 30 minutes, or up to overnight, before cooking.
- For a hotter meal, add a pinch of cayenne pepper to the marinade.
- Serve with a dish of Mexican rice or black beans.

MEDITERRANEAN STEAK SANDWICHES

- **Prep Time: 15 minutes**
- **Cooking Time: 10 minutes**
- **Serving Time: 5 minutes**

NUTRITIONAL VALUE (PER SERVING):

- Calories: 450
- Fat: 20g
- Saturated Fat: 5g
- Carbohydrates: 35g
- Fiber: 5g
- Sugar: 5g
- Protein: 30g

INGREDIENTS:

- 2 flank steaks, thinly cut against the grain (approximately 1/4-inch thick)
- 1 tablespoon olive oil
- Salt and pepper to taste
- 1 baguette, sliced into four pieces
- ½ cup prepared hummus
- 1/4 cup crumbled feta cheese
- ¼ cup chopped red onion
- 2 teaspoons chopped fresh parsley

INSTRUCTIONS:

1. Pat the cut flank steaks dry with paper towels and season with salt and pepper.
2. Heat the olive oil in a large pan over medium-high heat.
3. Add the beef mixture and heat for 5-7 minutes, or until the meat is cooked through.
4. To construct the sandwiches, spread hummus over the bottom half of the baguette slices.
5. Top with sliced steak, crumbled feta cheese, sliced red onion, and chopped parsley.
6. Serve immediately.

Tips:

- For a more delicious sandwich, marinate the sliced beef in a combination of olive oil, lemon juice, oregano, and garlic powder for at least 30 minutes, or up to overnight, before cooking.
- For a hotter sandwich, add a sprinkle of red pepper flakes to the marinade.

- Serve with a side of Greek salad or roasted veggies.

ROASTED BEEF WITH PEPPERCORN SAUCE

- **Prep Time: 20 minutes**
- **Cooking Time: 40 minutes**
- **Serving Time: 5 minutes**

NUTRITIONAL VALUE (PER SERVING):

- Calories: 350
- Fat: 20g
- Saturated Fat: 5g
- Carbohydrates: 10g
- Fiber: 2g
- Sugar: 5g
- Protein: 35g

INGREDIENTS:

- 2 pounds' beef tenderloin roast
- 1 tablespoon olive oil
- Salt and pepper to taste
- 2 teaspoons crushed black peppercorns
- 1/2 cup beef broth
- 1/4 cup heavy cream

INSTRUCTIONS:

1. Preheat oven to 325 degrees F (165 degrees C).
2. Pat the beef tenderloin roast dry with paper towels and season with salt and pepper.
3. Heat the olive oil in a large pan over medium-high heat.
4. Sear the beef tenderloin roast on all sides until browned, approximately 5 minutes each side.
5. Transfer the beef tenderloin roast to a roasting pan and roast for 20-25 minutes, or until the internal temperature hits 145 degrees F (63 degrees C) for medium-rare.
6. Remove the beef tenderloin roast from the oven and allow rest for 10 minutes before slicing.
7. To prepare the sauce, mix together the crushed black peppercorns and beef stock in a small saucepan.
8. Bring to a boil and cook for 5 minutes, or until the sauce has thickened.
9. Stir in the heavy cream and simmer for 1 minute longer.
10. Slice the beef tenderloin roast and serve with the peppercorn sauce.

Tip:

- For more savory dinner, serve the roasted beef with a side of roasted vegetables, such as carrots, parsnips, or Brussels sprouts.

- Prep Time: 20 minutes
- Marinating Time: 2 hours
- Cooking Time: 10 minutes
- Serving Time: 5 minutes

NUTRITIONAL VALUE (PER SERVING):

- Calories: 300
- Fat: 15g
- Saturated Fat: 4g
- Carbohydrates: 5g
- Fiber: 1g
- Sugar: 2g
- Protein: 35g

INGREDIENTS:

- 2 flank steaks (approximately 1-pound total)
- 1/4 cup strong brewed coffee
- 2 tablespoons olive oil
- 1 tablespoon soy sauce
- 1 teaspoon dried oregano
- 1 teaspoon dried thyme
- 1/2 teaspoon salt
- 1/4 teaspoon black pepper

INSTRUCTIONS:

1. In a large bowl, stir together the coffee, olive oil, soy sauce, oregano, thyme, salt, and pepper.
2. Add the flank steaks to the marinade and toss to coat.
3. Cover and refrigerate for at least 2 hours, or up to overnight.
4. Preheat oven to 400 degrees F (200 degrees C).
5. Remove the flank steaks from the marinade and discard the marinade.
6. Heat a large skillet over medium-high heat.
7. Add the flank steaks and heat for 3-4 minutes each side, or until browned and cooked through.
8. Let rest for 5 minutes before slicing.
9. Serve immediately.

Tip:

- For more savory dinner, serve the coffee-and-herb-marinated steak with a side of roasted vegetables, such as asparagus, zucchini, or bell peppers.

TRADITIONAL BEEF STROGANOFF

- Prep Time: 20 minutes
- Cooking Time: 15 minutes
- Serving Time: 5 minutes

NUTRITIONAL VALUE (PER SERVING):

- Calories: 350

- Fat: 20g
- Saturated Fat: 5g
- Carbohydrates: 15g
- Fiber: 2g
- Sugar: 5g
- Protein: 30g

INGREDIENTS:

- 1-pound beef sirloin, thinly sliced
- 1 tablespoon olive oil
- 1 onion, thinly sliced
- 2 tablespoons all-purpose flour
- 2 cups beef broth
- 1/2 cup sour cream
- 1 tablespoon Worcestershire sauce
- 1 tablespoon Dijon mustard
- 1/2 teaspoon salt
- 1/4 teaspoon black pepper

INSTRUCTIONS:

1. In a large bowl, mix the sliced beef sirloin, olive oil, and salt.
2. Toss to coat and put aside.
3. Heat the olive oil in a large pan over medium-high heat.
4. Add the sliced onion and simmer until softened, approximately 5 minutes.
5. Sprinkle the flour over the onions and heat for 1 minute, stirring frequently.
6. Gradually whisk in the beef broth until smooth.
7. Bring to a boil and cook for 5 minutes, or until the sauce has thickened.
8. Stir in the sour cream, Worcestershire sauce, Dijon mustard, salt, and pepper.
9. Add the cooked meat and any residual juices to the sauce.
10. Cook until heated thoroughly, approximately 2 minutes.
11. Serve immediately over egg noodles or rice.

Tips:

- For more savory stroganoff, prepare your own beef broth using cattle bones and veggies.
- For a richer stroganoff, add full-fat sour cream.
- If the sauce is too thick, add a bit more beef broth. If the sauce is too thin, boil for a few more minutes until thickened.
- Garnish with chopped fresh parsley.

CHICKEN AND ROASTED VEGETABLE WRAPS

- Prep Time: 15 minutes
- Cooking Time: 30 minutes
- Serving Time: 5 minutes

NUTRITIONAL VALUE (PER SERVING):

- Calories: 300
- Fat: 15g
- Saturated Fat: 4g
- Carbohydrates: 25g
- Fiber: 3g
- Sugar: 5g
- Protein: 20g

INGREDIENTS:

- 1 pound boneless, skinless chicken breasts
- 1 tablespoon olive oil
- Salt and pepper to taste
- 1 cup roasted veggies, such as carrots, zucchini, and bell peppers
- 4 large tortillas

INSTRUCTIONS:

1. Preheat oven to 400 degrees F (200 degrees C).
2. Toss the veggies with olive oil, salt, and pepper.
3. Spread the veggies on a baking sheet and roast for 20 minutes, or until soft.
4. In a large pan, heat the olive oil over medium-high heat.
5. Add the chicken breasts and heat for 5-7 minutes each side, or until cooked through.
6. Slice the chicken breasts.
7. To construct the wraps, cover each tortilla with a dab of hummus.
8. Top with roasted veggies, sliced chicken, and a sprinkling of chopped fresh parsley.
9. Roll up the wraps and enjoy.

Tip:

- For more savory wrap, add a dollop of sour cream or guacamole to each wrap.

SPICY CHICKEN CACCIATORE

- **Prep Time: 20 minutes**
- **Cooking Time: 30 minutes**
- **Serving Time: 5 minutes**

NUTRITIONAL VALUE (PER SERVING):

- Calories: 350
- Fat: 15g
- Saturated Fat: 4g
- Carbohydrates: 25g
- Fiber: 3g
- Sugar: 5g
- Protein: 30g

INGREDIENTS:

- 1 pound boneless, skinless chicken thighs, sliced into bite-sized pieces
- 1 tablespoon olive oil
- Salt and pepper to taste
- 1 onion, chopped
- 2 cloves garlic, minced

- 1 green bell pepper, chopped
- 1 red bell pepper, chopped
- 1 (14.5-ounce) can chopped tomatoes, undrained
- 1/2 cup chicken broth
- 1 teaspoon dried oregano
- 1/2 teaspoon crushed red pepper flakes

INSTRUCTIONS:

1. In a large pan, heat the olive oil over medium-high heat.
2. Add the chicken and heat until browned on both sides, approximately 5 minutes.
3. Season with salt and pepper.
4. Remove the chicken from the skillet and put aside.
5. Add the onion and garlic to the pan and simmer until softened, approximately 5 minutes.
6. Add the green bell pepper, red bell pepper, chopped tomatoes, chicken broth, oregano, and red pepper flakes.
7. Bring to a simmer and cook for 10 minutes.
8. Return the chicken to the skillet and cook for 5 minutes longer, or until cooked through.
9. Serve over spaghetti or rice.

Tip:

- For a hotter cacciatore, add additional crushed red pepper flakes to taste.

CHICKEN WITH CREAMY THYME SAUCE

- **Prep Time: 15 minutes**
- **Cooking Time: 20 minutes**
- **Serving Time: 5 minutes**

NUTRITIONAL VALUE (PER SERVING):

- Calories: 350
- Fat: 15g
- Saturated Fat: 5g
- Carbohydrates: 20g
- Fiber: 2g
- Sugar: 5g
- Protein: 30g

INGREDIENTS:

- 4 boneless, skinless chicken breasts
- 1 tablespoon olive oil
- Salt and pepper to taste
- 1 tablespoon butter
- 1 onion, chopped
- 2 cloves garlic, minced
- 1/4 cup chicken broth
- 1/4 cup heavy cream
- 1 tablespoon fresh thyme leaves
- 1/4 teaspoon lemon juice

INSTRUCTIONS:

1. In a large pan, heat the olive oil over medium-high heat.

2. Add the chicken breasts and heat for 5-7 minutes each side, or until cooked through.

3. Season with salt and pepper.

4. Remove the chicken from the skillet and put aside.

5. Melt the butter in the skillet.

6. Add the onion and simmer until softened, approximately 5 minutes.

7. Add the garlic and heat for 30 seconds longer, until fragrant.

8. Stir in the chicken broth, heavy cream, thyme leaves, and lemon juice.

9. Bring to a boil and cook for 5 minutes, or until the sauce has thickened.

10. Return the chicken to the pan and coat with the sauce.

11. Serve immediately.

Tip:

- For more savory dinner, serve the chicken with a side of roasted vegetables, such as carrots, parsnips, or Brussels sprouts.

ONE-POT ROASTED CHICKEN DINNER

- Prep Time: 20 minutes
- Cooking Time: 1 hour
- Serving Time: 10 minutes

NUTRITIONAL VALUE (PER SERVING):

- Calories: 400
- Fat: 20g
- Saturated Fat: 5g
- Carbohydrates: 30g
- Fiber: 3g
- Sugar: 5g
- Protein: 35g

INGREDIENTS:

- 1 entire chicken, chopped into pieces
- 1 tablespoon olive oil
- Salt and pepper to taste
- 1 onion, chopped
- 2 carrots, chopped
- 2 potatoes, chopped
- 1 cup chicken broth
- 1/4 cup heavy cream

INSTRUCTIONS:

1. Preheat oven to 400 degrees F (200 degrees C).

2. In a large bowl, mix the chicken pieces with olive oil, salt, and pepper.

3. Transfer the chicken to a roasting pan.

4. Add the onion, carrots, and potatoes to the roasting pan.

5. Pour the chicken stock over the chicken and veggies.

6. Roast for 1 hour, or until the chicken is cooked through and the veggies are soft.

7. Stir in the heavy cream and serve immediately.

Tip:

- For more savory meal, add a few sprigs of fresh herbs, such as thyme or rosemary, to the roasting pan before cooking.

🍄 MUSHROOMS WITH BELL PEPPERS

- **Prep Time: 10 minutes**
- **Cooking Time: 10 minutes**
- **Serving Time: 5 minutes**

NUTRITIONAL VALUE (PER SERVING):

- Calories: 100
- Fat: 5g
- Saturated Fat: 1g
- Carbohydrates: 10g
- Fiber: 2g
- Sugar: 5g
- Protein: 5g

INGREDIENTS:

- 1 tablespoon olive oil
- 1 onion, thinly sliced
- 1 green bell pepper, finely sliced
- 1 red bell pepper, thinly sliced
- 8 ounces sliced mushrooms
- Salt and pepper to taste

INSTRUCTIONS:

1. Heat the olive oil in a large pan over medium-high heat.

2. Add the onion and simmer until softened, approximately 5 minutes.

3. Add the green bell pepper, red bell pepper, and mushrooms.

4. Cook until the peppers are soft and the mushrooms are browned, approximately 5 minutes.

5. Season with salt and pepper.

6. Serve immediately.

Tip:

- For a more delicious meal, add a splash of balsamic vinegar or soy sauce to the pan before serving.

BELL PEPPERS & TOMATO CASSEROLE

- **Prep Time: 15 minutes**
- **Cooking Time: 45 minutes**
- **Serving Time: 10 minutes**

NUTRITIONAL VALUE (PER SERVING):

- Calories: 250
- Fat: 10g
- Saturated Fat: 2g
- Carbohydrates: 30g
- Fiber: 5g
- Sugar: 10g
- Protein: 10g

INGREDIENTS:

- 2 tablespoons olive oil
- 1 onion, chopped
- 2 cloves garlic, minced
- 2 green bell peppers, chopped
- 2 red bell peppers, chopped
- 1 (14.5-ounce) can chopped tomatoes, undrained
- 1/2 cup tomato sauce
- 1/4 cup chopped fresh parsley
- 1 teaspoon dried oregano
- 1/2 teaspoon salt
- 1/4 teaspoon black pepper
- 1 cup shredded Monterey Jack cheese

INSTRUCTIONS:

1. Preheat oven to 350 degrees F (175 degrees C).
2. Heat the olive oil in a large pan over medium heat.
3. Add the onion and simmer until softened, approximately 5 minutes.
4. Add the garlic and heat for 30 seconds longer, until fragrant.
5. Add the green bell peppers, red bell peppers, chopped tomatoes, tomato sauce, parsley, oregano, salt, and pepper.
6. Bring to a boil and cook for 5 minutes.
7. Pour the mixture into a greased 9x13-inch baking dish.
8. Sprinkle the cheese over the top.
9. Bake for 30 minutes, or until the cheese is melted and bubbling.
10. Serve immediately.

Tip:

- For more savory casserole, add a cooked ground beef to the pan before adding the veggies.

VEGGIES CASSEROLE

- **Prep Time: 15 minutes**
- **Cooking Time: 45 minutes**
- **Serving Time: 10 minutes**

NUTRITIONAL VALUE (PER SERVING):

- Calories: 200
- Fat: 5g
- Saturated Fat: 1g
- Carbohydrates: 35g
- Fiber: 5g
- Sugar: 5g
- Protein: 5g

- 2 tablespoons olive oil
- 1 onion, chopped
- 2 cloves garlic, minced
- 1 zucchini, chopped
- 1 yellow squash, chopped
- 1 cup chopped broccoli florets
- 1 cup chopped cauliflower florets
- 1 (14.5-ounce) can chopped tomatoes, undrained
- 1/2 cup vegetable broth
- 1/4 cup grated Parmesan cheese
- 1 teaspoon dried oregano
- 1/2 teaspoon salt
- 1/4 teaspoon black pepper

INSTRUCTIONS:

1. Preheat oven to 350 degrees F (175 degrees C).
2. Heat the olive oil in a large pan over medium heat.
3. Add the onion and simmer until softened, approximately 5 minutes.
4. Add the garlic and heat for 30 seconds longer, until fragrant.
5. Add the zucchini, yellow squash, broccoli, cauliflower, chopped tomatoes, vegetable broth, Parmesan cheese, oregano, salt, and pepper.
6. Bring to a boil and cook for 5 minutes.
7. Pour the mixture into a greased 9x13-inch baking dish.
8. Bake for 30 minutes, or until the veggies are soft and the casserole is bubbling.
9. Serve immediately.

Tip:

- For more savory casserole, top with a dab of sour cream or Greek yogurt.

SWEET & SPICY CHICKPEAS

- **Prep Time: 10 minutes**
- **Cooking Time: 15 minutes**
- **Serving Time: 5 minutes**

NUTRITIONAL VALUE (PER SERVING):

- Calories: 300
- Fat: 10g
- Saturated Fat: 2g
- Carbohydrates: 40g
- Fiber: 8g
- Sugar: 10g
- Protein: 15g

INGREDIENTS:

- 1 (15-ounce) can chickpeas, drained and rinsed
- 1 tablespoon olive oil
- 1 tablespoon honey
- 1 teaspoon sriracha sauce
- 1/2 teaspoon cumin

- 1/4 teaspoon salt
- 1/4 teaspoon black pepper

INSTRUCTIONS:

1. Preheat oven to 400 degrees F (200 degrees C).
2. Line a baking sheet with parchment paper.
3. In a large bowl, mix the chickpeas, olive oil, honey, sriracha sauce, cumin, salt, and pepper.
4. Toss to coat evenly.
5. Spread the chickpeas on the prepared baking sheet.
6. Bake for 15 minutes, or until the chickpeas are crispy.
7. Serve immediately.

Tip:

- For more savory snack, add a sprinkling of chopped fresh parsley or cilantro.

CHICKPEAS & VEGGIE STEW

- Prep Time: 20 minutes
- Cooking Time: 30 minutes
- Serving Time: 5 minutes

NUTRITIONAL VALUE (PER SERVING):

- Calories: 350
- Fat: 15g
- Saturated Fat: 3g
- Carbohydrates: 45g
- Fiber: 10g
- Sugar: 5g
- Protein: 20g

INGREDIENTS:

- 1 tablespoon olive oil
- 1 onion, chopped 2 cloves garlic, minced
- 1 (14.5-ounce) can chopped tomatoes, undrained
- 1 (15-ounce) can chickpeas, drained and rinsed
- 1 cup vegetarian broth 1/2 cup chopped carrots
- 1/2 cup sliced celery 1 teaspoon dry oregano
- 1/2 teaspoon salt 1/4 teaspoon black pepper

INSTRUCTIONS:

1. Heat the olive oil in a big saucepan over medium heat.
2. Add the onion and simmer until softened, approximately 5 minutes.
3. Add the garlic and heat for 30 seconds longer, until fragrant.

4. Stir in the chopped tomatoes, chickpeas, vegetable broth, carrots, celery, oregano, salt, and pepper.

5. Bring to a boil and cook for 20 minutes, or until the veggies are cooked.

6. Serve immediately.

Tip:

- For a savory stew, add a dash of red wine vinegar or balsamic vinegar before serving.

ALMOND-CRUSTED SALMON

- **Prep Time: 15 minutes**
- **Cooking Time: 20 minutes**
- **Serving Time: 5 minutes**

NUTRITIONAL VALUE (PER SERVING):

- Calories: 400
- Fat: 20g
- Saturated Fat: 4g
- Carbohydrates: 5g
- Fiber: 1g
- Sugar: 5g
- Protein: 35g

INGREDIENTS:

- 2 (4-ounce) salmon fillets
- 1/4 cup sliced almonds
- 1 tablespoon olive oil
- 1/2 teaspoon salt
- 1/4 teaspoon black pepper

INSTRUCTIONS:

1. Preheat oven to 400 degrees F (200 degrees C).

2. Line a baking sheet with parchment paper.

3. In a small bowl, add the sliced almonds, olive oil, salt, and pepper.

4. Press the almond mixture onto the salmon fillets, covering evenly.

5. Place the salmon fillets on the prepared baking sheet.

6. Bake for 15-20 minutes, or until the salmon is cooked through and the almonds are golden brown.

7. Serve immediately.

Tip:

- For a savory dinner, serve the almond-crusted salmon with a side of roasted vegetables, such as asparagus, broccoli, or Brussels sprouts.

CHICKEN & VEGGIE BOWL WITH BROWN RICE

- **Prep Time: 20 minutes**
- **Cooking Time: 30 minutes**
- **Serving Time: 5 minutes**

- Calories: 450
- Fat: 20g
- Saturated Fat: 5g
- Carbohydrates: 45g
- Fiber: 5g
- Sugar: 5g
- Protein: 40g

INGREDIENTS:

- 1 cup cooked brown rice
- 1 tablespoon olive oil
- 1 boneless, skinless chicken breast, cooked and shredded
- 1 cup broccoli florets, cooked
- 1/2 cup carrots, diced and cooked
- 1/4 cup red bell pepper, chopped
- 1/4 cup chopped green onions
- 2 teaspoons low-sodium soy sauce

INSTRUCTIONS:

1. Divide the cooked brown rice equally among four bowls.
2. In a large skillet, heat the olive oil over medium heat.
3. Add the shredded chicken, broccoli florets, diced carrots, red bell pepper, and sliced green onions.
4. Cook for 5-7 minutes, or until the veggies are soft.
5. Stir in the low-sodium soy sauce.
6. Divide the chicken and vegetable mixture equally among the bowls of rice.
7. Serve immediately.

BEEF STEAK FAJITAS

- **Prep Time: 15 minutes**
- **Cooking Time: 10 minutes**
- **Serving Time: 5 minutes**

NUTRITIONAL VALUE (PER SERVING):

- Calories: 400
- Fat: 20g
- Saturated Fat: 7g
- Carbohydrates: 35g
- Fiber: 5g
- Sugar: 5g
- Protein: 30g

INGREDIENTS:

- 1-pound flank steak, thinly cut against the grain (approximately 1/4-inch thick)
- 1 tablespoon olive oil
- 1 onion, thinly sliced
- 1 green bell pepper, finely sliced
- 1 red bell pepper, thinly sliced
- 1 tablespoon chili powder
- 1 teaspoon ground cumin
- 1/2 teaspoon salt

- 1/4 teaspoon black pepper

INSTRUCTIONS:

1. In a large bowl, mix the sliced flank steak, olive oil, onion, green bell pepper, red bell pepper, chili powder, cumin, salt, and pepper.
2. Toss to coat evenly.
3. Heat a large skillet over medium-high heat.
4. Add the meat mixture and heat for 5-7 minutes, or until the steak is cooked through and the veggies are soft.
5. Serve immediately with warm tortillas, your favorite toppings, such as shredded cheese, sour cream, guacamole, and salsa.

ITALIAN PORK CHOPS

- **Prep Time: 20 minutes**
- **Cooking Time: 15 minutes**
- **Serving Time: 5 minutes**

NUTRITIONAL VALUE (PER SERVING):

- Calories: 350
- Fat: 15g
- Saturated Fat: 4g
- Carbohydrates: 15g
- Fiber: 2g
- Sugar: 5g
- Protein: 30g

INGREDIENTS:

- 4 bone-in pork chops
- 1 tablespoon olive oil
- 1/2 teaspoon salt 1/4 teaspoon black pepper
- 1/4 cup Italian dressing
- 2 cloves garlic, minced

INSTRUCTIONS:

1. Preheat oven to 400 degrees F (200 degrees C).
2. In a large bowl, mix the pork chops, olive oil, salt, and pepper.
3. Toss to coat evenly.
4. Place the pork chops in a baking dish.
5. Pour the Italian dressing over the pork chops.
6. Sprinkle the garlic on top of the pork chops.
7. Bake for 15-20 minutes, or until the pork chops are cooked through and no longer pink in the middle.
8. Serve immediately.

Tip:

- For a savory dinner, serve the Italian pork chops with a side of pasta or rice.

CHICKEN MUSHROOM STROGANOFF

- **Prep Time: 15 minutes**
- **Cooking Time: 20 minutes**
- **Serving Time: 5 minutes**

NUTRITIONAL VALUE (PER SERVING):

- Calories: 400
- Fat: 20g
- Saturated Fat: 5g
- Carbohydrates: 25g
- Fiber: 3g
- Sugar: 5g
- Protein: 30g

INGREDIENTS:

- 1 tablespoon olive oil
- 1 onion, thinly sliced 8 ounces' mushrooms, sliced 1 pound boneless, skinless chicken breasts, chopped into bite-sized pieces
- 1 tablespoon paprika
- 1 teaspoon Dijon mustard
- 1/2 cup sour cream
- 1/4 cup beef broth 1/4 teaspoon salt
- 1/4 teaspoon black pepper

INSTRUCTIONS:

1. In a large skillet, heat the olive oil over medium heat.
2. Add the onion and simmer until softened, approximately 5 minutes.
3. Add the mushrooms and heat until browned, approximately 5 minutes.
4. Add the chicken, paprika, and Dijon mustard.
5. Cook until the chicken is browned and cooked through, approximately 5 minutes.
6. Stir in the sour cream, beef broth, salt, and pepper.
7. Bring to a boil and cook for 5 minutes, or until the sauce has thickened.
8. Serve immediately over egg noodles or rice.

GRILLED TUNA KEBABS

- **Prep Time: 15 minutes**
- **Cooking Time: 10 minutes**
- **Serving Time: 5 minutes**

NUTRITIONAL VALUE (PER SERVING):

- Calories: 250
- Fat: 10g
- Saturated Fat: 2g
- Carbohydrates: 5g
- Fiber: 1g
- Sugar: 5g
- Protein: 30g

INGREDIENTS:

- 1-pound tuna steaks, cut into 1-inch cubes
- 1 tablespoon olive oil
- 1 lemon, juiced and zested
- 1 teaspoon dried oregano
- 1/2 teaspoon salt
- 1/4 teaspoon black pepper
- 1 red bell pepper, sliced into 1-inch pieces
- 1 zucchini, sliced into 1-inch chunks

INSTRUCTIONS:

1. In a large bowl, mix the tuna cubes, olive oil, lemon juice, lemon zest, oregano, salt, and pepper.
2. Toss to coat evenly.
3. Thread the tuna cubes, red bell pepper pieces, and zucchini pieces onto skewers.
4. Preheat grill or grill pan to medium-high heat.
5. Grill the skewers for 5-7 minutes each side, or until the tuna is cooked through and the veggies are soft.
6. Serve immediately with your favorite dipping sauce, such as marinara sauce or tzatziki sauce.

CAST IRON PORK LOIN

- **Prep Time: 20 minutes**
- **Cooking Time: 30 minutes**
- **Serving Time: 5 minutes**

NUTRITIONAL VALUE (PER SERVING):

- Calories: 450
- Fat: 25g
- Saturated Fat: 7g
- Carbohydrates: 3g
- Fiber: 1g
- Sugar: 2g
- Protein: 40g

INGREDIENTS:

- 1 pound boneless, skinless pork loin roast
- 1 tablespoon olive oil 1/2 teaspoon salt 1/4 teaspoon black pepper
- 1 tablespoon Dijon mustard
- 1 tablespoon honey
- 1 teaspoon dried thyme

INSTRUCTIONS:

- Preheat oven to 375 degrees F (190 degrees C).
- In a small bowl, mix together the Dijon mustard, honey, and thyme.
- Remove the silver skin from the pork loin roast.
- Rub the pork loin roast with the olive oil, salt, and pepper.
- Spread the Honey-Dijon mixture evenly over the pork loin roast.

- Place the pork loin roast in a cast iron pan.

- Transfer the pan to the oven and roast for 25-30 minutes, or until the pork loin roast is cooked through and reaches an internal temperature of 145 degrees F (63 degrees C).

- Let the pork loin rest for 5 minutes before slicing and serving.

CRISPY BAKED TOFU

- **Prep Time: 15 minutes**
- **Cooking Time: 25 minutes**
- **Serving Time: 5 minutes**

NUTRITIONAL VALUE (PER SERVING):

- Calories: 200
- Fat: 10g
- Saturated Fat: 2g
- Carbohydrates: 10g
- Fiber: 5g
- Sugar: 0g
- Protein: 15g

INGREDIENTS:

- 1 (14-ounce) block extra-firm tofu, rinsed and patted dry
- 1 tablespoon cornstarch
- 1 tablespoon olive oil
- 1/2 teaspoon salt
- 1/4 teaspoon black pepper

INSTRUCTIONS:

1. Preheat oven to 400 degrees F (200 degrees C).
2. Cut the tofu into 1-inch pieces.
3. In a large dish, mix the tofu cubes with the cornstarch, olive oil, salt, and pepper until equally covered.
4. Spread the tofu cubes in a single layer on a baking sheet coated with parchment paper.
5. Bake for 25 minutes, or until the tofu is golden brown and crispy.
6. Serve immediately with your favorite dipping sauce, such as soy sauce, sweet chili sauce, or sriracha mayo.

ROASTED TOMATO BRUSSELS SPROUTS

- **Prep Time: 10 minutes**
- **Cooking Time: 20 minutes**
- **Serving Time: 5 minutes**

NUTRITIONAL VALUE (PER SERVING):

- Calories: 50
- Fat: 3g
- Saturated Fat: 0g
- Carbohydrates: 10g
- Fiber: 4g

- Sugar: 5g
- Protein: 2g

INGREDIENTS:

- 1 pound Brussels sprouts, trimmed and halved
- 1 tablespoon olive oil
- 1/2 teaspoon salt
- 1/4 teaspoon black pepper
- 1 roma tomato, chopped

INSTRUCTIONS:

1. Preheat oven to 400 degrees F (200 degrees C) and line a baking sheet with parchment paper.
2. In a large bowl, mix the Brussels sprouts, olive oil, salt, and pepper until equally covered.
3. Spread the Brussels sprouts in a single layer on the prepared baking sheet.
4. Add the diced roma tomato to the baking sheet.
5. Roast for 20 minutes, or until the Brussels sprouts are tender and golden brown.
6. Serve immediately.

Tips:

- For a savory side dish, add a sprinkling of grated Parmesan cheese or balsamic glaze before serving.
- To make the Brussels sprouts extremely crispy, roast them for an additional 5-10 minutes.
- For a more colorful meal, add a dash of red wine vinegar or lemon juice before serving.

SIMPLE SAUTÉED GREENS

- **Prep Time: 5 minutes**
- **Cooking Time: 5 minutes**
- **Serving Time: 5 minutes**

NUTRITIONAL VALUE (PER SERVING):

- Calories: 30
- Fat: 1g
- Saturated Fat: 0g
- Carbohydrates: 5g
- Fiber: 2g
- Sugar: 2g
- Protein: 2g

INGREDIENTS:

- 1 bunch leafy green vegetables, such as kale, spinach, or collard greens, stemmed and washed
- 1 tablespoon olive oil
- Salt and pepper to taste

INSTRUCTIONS:

1. Heat the olive oil in a large pan over medium heat.

2. Add the leafy green veggies and simmer for 5 minutes, or until wilted.

3. Season with salt and pepper to taste.

4. Serve immediately.

GARLICKY MUSHROOMS

- Prep Time: 5 minutes
- Cooking Time: 10 minutes
- Serving Time: 5 minutes

NUTRITIONAL VALUE (PER SERVING):

- Calories: 60
- Fat: 3g
- Saturated Fat: 1g
- Carbohydrates: 5g
- Fiber: 2g
- Sugar: 2g
- Protein: 3g

INGREDIENTS:

- 8 ounces' mushrooms, sliced
- 1 tablespoon olive oil
- 2 cloves garlic, minced
- Salt and pepper to taste

INSTRUCTIONS:

1. Heat the olive oil in a large pan over medium heat.

2. Add the mushrooms and simmer for 5 minutes, or until tender.

3. Add the garlic and heat for 30 seconds longer, until fragrant.

4. Season with salt and pepper to taste.

5. Serve immediately.

Tips:

- For a savory side dish, add a sprinkling of chopped fresh parsley or chives before serving.

- To add a touch of richness, add a tablespoon of butter or ghee to the pan before cooking the mushrooms.

- For a spicy touch, add a sprinkle of red pepper flakes to the pan along with the garlic.

GREEN BEANS IN OVEN

- Prep Time: 10 minutes
- Cooking Time: 15 minutes
- Serving Time: 5 minutes

NUTRITIONAL VALUE (PER SERVING):

- Calories: 40
- Fat: 2g
- Saturated Fat: 0g
- Carbohydrates: 7g
- Fiber: 3g
- Sugar: 2g

Protein: 2g

INGREDIENTS:

- 1 pound fresh green beans, trimmed
- 1 tablespoon olive oil
- Salt and pepper to taste

INSTRUCTIONS:

1. Preheat oven to 400 degrees F (200 degrees C) and line a baking sheet with parchment paper.
2. In a large bowl, mix the green beans, olive oil, salt, and pepper until equally covered.
3. Spread the green beans in a single layer on the prepared baking sheet.
4. Roast for 15 minutes, or until the green beans are soft and crisp.
5. Serve immediately.

CAULIFLOWER RICE

- **Prep Time: 10 minutes**
- **Cooking Time: 10 minutes**
- **Serving Time: 5 minutes**

NUTRITIONAL VALUE (PER SERVING):

- Calories: 25
- Fat: 1g
- Saturated Fat: 0g
- Carbohydrates: 5g
- Fiber: 2g
- Sugar: 2g
- Protein: 2g

INGREDIENTS:

- 1 head of cauliflower, trimmed and florets removed
- 1 tablespoon olive oil
- Salt and pepper to taste

INSTRUCTIONS:

1. In a food processor, pulse the cauliflower florets until they resemble rice.
2. Heat the olive oil in a large pan over medium heat.
3. Add the cauliflower rice and simmer for 5 minutes, or until softened.
4. Season with salt and pepper to taste.
5. Serve immediately.

Tips:

- For a more flavored cauliflower rice, add a sprinkle of turmeric, cumin, or curry powder before cooking.
- To add extra nutrients, combine the cauliflower rice with cooked quinoa or brown rice.
- For a richer meal, add a tablespoon of butter or ghee to the pan before cooking the cauliflower rice.

AIR-FRIED BRUSSELS SPROUTS

- Prep Time: 10 minutes
- Cooking Time: 15 minutes
- Serving Time: 5 minutes

NUTRITIONAL VALUE (PER SERVING):

- Calories: 50
- Fat: 3g
- Saturated Fat: 0g
- Carbohydrates: 10g
- Fiber: 4g
- Sugar: 5g
- Protein: 2g

INGREDIENTS:

- 1 pound Brussels sprouts, trimmed and halved
- 1 tablespoon olive oil
- Salt and pepper to taste

INSTRUCTIONS:

1. Preheat air fryer to 400 degrees F (200 degrees C).
2. In a large bowl, mix the Brussels sprouts, olive oil, salt, and pepper until equally covered.
3. Spread the Brussels sprouts in a single layer in the air fryer basket.
4. Cook for 15 minutes, or until the Brussels sprouts are soft and golden brown.
5. Serve immediately.

Tips:

- For extra crispy Brussels sprouts, jiggle the air fryer basket halfway through cooking.
- To add extra flavor, mix the Brussels sprouts with a tablespoon of balsamic glaze before air fried.
- For a bit of richness, add a sprinkle of grated Parmesan cheese before serving.
- Additional Tips for Roasted Tomato Brussels Sprouts
- For a smokier taste, roast the Brussels sprouts with a couple cloves of garlic and a sprig of rosemary.
- To add a touch of sweetness, sprinkle the Brussels sprouts with honey or maple syrup before roasting.
- For a spicy kick, add a sprinkle of red pepper flakes to the baking sheet before roasting.

ROSEMARY POTATOES

- Prep Time: 10 minutes
- Cooking Time: 30 minutes
- Serving Time: 5 minutes

NUTRITIONAL VALUE (PER SERVING):

- Calories: 250
- Fat: 10g
- Saturated Fat: 2g
- Carbohydrates: 35g
- Fiber: 3g
- Sugar: 2g
- Protein: 3g

INGREDIENTS:

- 1 pound new potatoes, halved
- 2 tablespoons olive oil
- 1 teaspoon dried rosemary
- 1/2 teaspoon salt
- 1/4 teaspoon black pepper

INSTRUCTIONS:

1. Preheat oven to 400 degrees F (200 degrees C).
2. In a large basin, combine the potatoes, olive oil, rosemary, salt, and pepper until equally covered.
3. Spread the potatoes in a single layer on a baking sheet coated with parchment paper.
4. Roast for 30 minutes, or until the potatoes are soft and golden brown.
5. Serve immediately.

Tips:

- For extra crispy potatoes, roast them for an additional 5-10 minutes.
- To add extra flavor, sprinkle the potatoes with a tablespoon of balsamic glaze before roasting.
- For a bit of richness, add a sprinkle of grated Parmesan cheese before serving.

CORN ON THE COB

- **Prep Time: 5 minutes**
- **Cooking Time: 10 minutes**
- **Serving Time: 5 minutes**

NUTRITIONAL VALUE (PER SERVING):

- Calories: 100
- Fat: 3g
- Saturated Fat: 1g
- Carbohydrates: 20g
- Fiber: 2g
- Sugar: 3g
- Protein: 4g

INGREDIENTS:

- 4 ears of corn, husked

INSTRUCTIONS:

1. Bring a big saucepan of salted water to a boil.

2. Add the corn and simmer for 10 minutes, or until cooked.

3. Drain and serve immediately.

CHILI LIME SALMON

- Prep Time: 10 minutes
- Cooking Time: 15 minutes
- Serving Time: 5 minutes

NUTRITIONAL VALUE (PER SERVING):

- Calories: 400
- Fat: 25g
- Saturated Fat: 5g
- Carbohydrates: 2g
- Fiber: 1g
- Sugar: 1g
- Protein: 35g

INGREDIENTS:

1. 2 salmon fillets (approximately 6 ounces each)
2. 1 tablespoon chili powder
3. 1 teaspoon lime juice
4. 1/2 teaspoon salt
5. 1/4 teaspoon black pepper

INSTRUCTIONS:

1. Preheat oven to 400 degrees F (200 degrees C).

2. In a small bowl, stir together the chili powder, lime juice, salt, and pepper.

3. Place the salmon fillets on a baking pan lined with parchment paper.

4. Brush the salmon fillets with the chili-lime mixture.

5. Bake for 15-20 minutes, or until the salmon is cooked through and flakes readily with a fork.

6. Serve immediately.

Tips:

- For a hotter salmon, add additional chili powder to the mixture.
- To add extra flavor, marinate the salmon in the chili-lime sauce for 30 minutes before baking.
- For a bit of richness, serve the salmon with a dollop of sour cream or Greek yogurt.

COLLARD GREENS

- Prep Time: 15 minutes
- Cooking Time: 20 minutes
- Serving Time: 5 minutes

NUTRITIONAL VALUE (PER SERVING):

- Calories: 200
- Fat: 10g

- Saturated Fat: 2g
- Carbohydrates: 20g
- Fiber: 9g
- Sugar: 5g
- Protein: 4g

INGREDIENTS:

- 1-pound collard greens, stemmed and washed
- 1 tablespoon olive oil
- 1/2 teaspoon salt
- 1/4 teaspoon black pepper
- 1/4 cup red wine vinegar

INSTRUCTIONS:

1. Heat the olive oil in a large pan over medium heat.
2. Add the collard greens and simmer for 10 minutes, or until wilted.
3. Season with salt and pepper.
4. Stir in the red wine vinegar and simmer for 5 minutes longer, or until the vinegar has decreased.
5. Serve immediately.

Tips:

- For a smokier taste, sauté the collard greens with a couple pieces of bacon.
- To add extra flavor, top the collard greens with a sprinkling of chopped fresh parsley or chives.
- For a hint of richness, add a tablespoon of butter or ghee to the pan before cooking the collard

AROMATIC TOASTED PUMPKIN SEEDS

- **Prep Time: 10 minutes**
- **Cooking Time: 20 minutes**
- **Serving Time: 5 minutes**

NUTRITIONAL VALUE (PER SERVING):

- Calories: 150
- Fat: 10g
- Saturated Fat: 2g
- Carbohydrates: 5g
- Fiber: 2g
- Sugar: 2g
- Protein: 4g

INGREDIENTS:

- 1 cup pumpkin seeds, washed and rubbed dry
- 1 tablespoon olive oil
- 1 teaspoon salt
- 1/2 teaspoon ground cumin
- 1/4 teaspoon smoked paprika

INSTRUCTIONS:

1. Preheat oven to 300 degrees F (150 degrees C).

2. In a large bowl, combine the pumpkin seeds, olive oil, salt, cumin, and paprika until equally covered.

3. Spread the pumpkin seeds in a single layer on a baking sheet coated with parchment paper.

4. Bake for 20-25 minutes, or until the pumpkin seeds are golden brown and toasted.

5. Let cool fully before serving.

BACON-WRAPPED SHRIMP

- **Prep Time: 10 minutes**
- **Cooking Time: 15 minutes**
- **Serving Time: 5 minutes**

NUTRITIONAL VALUE (PER SERVING):

- Calories: 250
- Fat: 15g
- Saturated Fat: 5g
- Carbohydrates: 2g
- Fiber: 0g
- Sugar: 1g
- Protein: 20g

INGREDIENTS:

- 1-pound shrimp, peeled and deveined
- 8 pieces of bacon
- 1 tablespoon olive oil
- Salt and pepper to taste

INSTRUCTIONS:

1. Preheat oven to 400 degrees F (200 degrees C).

2. Wrap each shrimp with a piece of bacon.

3. In a large skillet, heat the olive oil over medium heat.

4. Cook the bacon-wrapped shrimp for 5 minutes each side, or until the bacon is crispy and the shrimp is cooked through.

5. Season with salt and pepper to taste.

6. Serve immediately.

Tips:

- For added flavor, marinate the shrimp in a combination of soy sauce, rice vinegar, and sesame oil for 30 minutes before wrapping them in bacon.

- To add extra sweetness, brush the bacon-wrapped shrimp with honey or maple syrup before baking.

- For a bit of richness, serve the bacon-wrapped shrimp with a dollop of sour cream or Greek yogurt.

CHEESY BROCCOLI BITES

- **Prep Time: 15 minutes**
- **Cooking Time: 15 minutes**
- **Serving Time: 5 minutes**

NUTRITIONAL VALUE (PER SERVING):

- Calories: 100
- Fat: 5g
- Saturated Fat: 2g
- Carbohydrates: 10g
- Fiber: 2g
- Sugar: 2g
- Protein: 5g

INGREDIENTS:

- 1 head of broccoli, florets chopped into bite-sized pieces
- 1/4 cup shredded cheddar cheese
- 1 tablespoon olive oil
- Salt and pepper to taste

INSTRUCTIONS:

1. Preheat oven to 400 degrees F (200 degrees C) and line a baking sheet with parchment paper.
2. In a large bowl, mix the broccoli florets with the cheese, olive oil, salt, and pepper until equally covered.
3. Spread the broccoli florets in a single layer on the prepared baking sheet.
4. Bake for 15 minutes, or until the broccoli is cooked and the cheese is melted and bubbling.
5. Serve immediately.

Tips:

- For more savory side dish, add a sprinkling of chopped fresh parsley or chives before serving.
- To make the broccoli bits extremely crispy, roast them for an additional 5-10 minutes.
- For a richer meal, add a tablespoon of butter or ghee to the broccoli florets before tossing them with the cheese and olive oil.

EASY CAPRESE SKEWERS

- **Prep Time: 10 minutes**
- **Cooking Time: 0 minutes**
- **Serving Time: 5 minutes**

NUTRITIONAL VALUE (PER SERVING):

- Calories: 75
- Fat: 5g
- Saturated Fat: 2g
- Carbohydrates: 5g
- Fiber: 1g
- Sugar: 3g

- Protein: 3g

INGREDIENTS:

- 1-pound cherry tomatoes
- 1 ball of mozzarella cheese, sliced into bite-sized portions
- 12 fresh basil leaves

INSTRUCTIONS:

1. Thread the cherry tomatoes, mozzarella cheese chunks, and basil leaves onto skewers.
2. Serve immediately.

Tips:

- For more savory side dish, sprinkle the skewers with balsamic vinegar or olive oil before serving.
- To add extra nutrition, garnish the skewers with a sprinkling of chopped fresh parsley or oregano.
- For a richer meal, add a dollop of sour cream or Greek yogurt before serving.

GRILLED TOFU WITH SESAME SEEDS

- **Prep Time: 15 minutes**
- **Cooking Time: 10 minutes**
- **Serving Time: 5 minutes**

NUTRITIONAL VALUE (PER SERVING):

- Calories: 200
- Fat: 10g
- Saturated Fat: 2g
- Carbohydrates: 5g
- Fiber: 2g
- Sugar: 2g
- Protein: 15g

INGREDIENTS:

- 1 block extra-firm tofu, drained and patted dry
- 1 tablespoon olive oil
- 1 tablespoon soy sauce
- 1 teaspoon sesame seeds

INSTRUCTIONS:

1. Preheat grill or grill pan to medium-high heat.
2. Cut the tofu into 1-inch pieces.
3. In a large bowl, mix the tofu cubes with the olive oil, soy sauce, and sesame seeds until equally covered.
4. Grill the tofu cubes for 5 minutes each side, or until golden brown and crispy.
5. Serve immediately.

Tips:

- For more savory side dish, add a sprinkling of chopped fresh scallions or cilantro before serving.
- To make the tofu extremely crispy, press it between two plates with a weight on top for 15 minutes before cutting it into cubes.

- For a richer meal, add a spoonful of honey or maple syrup to the tofu before grilling.

KALE CHIPS

- **Prep Time: 10 minutes**
- **Cooking Time: 15 minutes**
- **Serving Time: 5 minutes**

NUTRITIONAL VALUE (PER SERVING):

- Calories: 50
- Fat: 3g
- Saturated Fat: 0g
- Carbohydrates: 5g
- Fiber: 3g
- Sugar: 2g
- Protein: 2g

INGREDIENTS:

- 1 bunch kale, stems removed and leaves cut into bite-sized pieces
- 1 tablespoon olive oil
- Salt and pepper to taste

INSTRUCTIONS:

1. Preheat oven to 350 degrees F (175 degrees C) and line a baking sheet with parchment paper.
2. In a large bowl, mix the kale leaves with the olive oil, salt, and pepper until equally coated.
3. Spread the kale leaves in a single layer on the prepared baking sheet.
4. Bake for 15-20 minutes, or until the kale leaves are crispy and dry.
5. Let cool fully before serving.

Tips:

- For more savory side dish, add a sprinkle of nutritional yeast or grated Parmesan cheese before serving.
- To make the kale chips extremely crispy, bake them for an additional 5-10 minutes.
- For a richer meal, mix the kale leaves with a tablespoon of melted butter or ghee before baking.

SIMPLE DEVILED EGGS

- **Prep Time: 15 minutes**
- **Cooking Time: 12 minutes**
- **Serving Time: 5 minutes**

NUTRITIONAL VALUE (PER SERVING):

- Calories: 100
- Fat: 7g
- Saturated Fat: 4g
- Carbohydrates: 1g

- Fiber: 0g
- Sugar: 1g
- Protein: 6g

INGREDIENTS:

- 6 hard-boiled eggs
- 1/4 cup mayonnaise
- 1 tablespoon Dijon mustard
- 1 teaspoon paprika
- Salt and pepper to taste

INSTRUCTIONS:

1. Peel the hard-boiled eggs and gently cut them in half lengthwise.
2. Scoop out the yolks and set them in a medium bowl.
3. Mash the yolks with the mayonnaise, mustard, paprika, salt, and pepper until smooth.
4. Spoon the yolk mixture back into the egg whites.
5. Serve immediately or refrigerate for later.

Tips:

- For more savory filling, add a touch of cayenne pepper or a splash of spicy sauce.
- To make the deviled eggs extra creamy, add a spoonful of sour cream or Greek yogurt to the yolk mixture.

- For a more festive look, top the deviled eggs with a sprig of fresh parsley or a sprinkling of paprika.

SAUTÉED COLLARD GREENS AND CABBAGE

- **Prep Time: 10 minutes**
- **Cooking Time: 15 minutes**
- **Serving Time: 5 minutes**

NUTRITIONAL VALUE (PER SERVING):

- Calories: 200
- Fat: 10g
- Saturated Fat: 2g
- Carbohydrates: 15g
- Fiber: 5g
- Sugar: 5g
- Protein: 4g

INGREDIENTS:

- 1-pound collard greens, stemmed and washed
- 1/2 head of cabbage, shredded 1 tablespoon olive oil
- Salt and pepper to taste

INSTRUCTIONS:

1. Heat the olive oil in a large pan over medium heat.

2. Add the collard greens and cabbage and simmer for 10 minutes, or until wilted.

3. Season with salt and pepper to taste.

4. Serve immediately.

Tips:

- For a smokier taste, simmer the collard greens and cabbage with a couple pieces of bacon.

- To add extra flavor, top the collard greens and cabbage with a sprinkling of chopped fresh parsley or chives.

- For a touch of richness, add a tablespoon of butter or ghee to the pan before cooking the collard greens and cabbage.

ROASTED DELICATA SQUASH WITH THYME

- **Prep Time: 10 minutes**
- **Cooking Time: 20 minutes**
- **Serving Time: 5 minutes**

NUTRITIONAL VALUE (PER SERVING):

- Calories: 150
- Fat: 6g
- Saturated Fat: 1g
- Carbohydrates: 25g
- Fiber: 3g
- Sugar: 10g
- Protein: 3g

INGREDIENTS:

- 1 medium delicata squash, halved and seeded
- 1 tablespoon olive oil
- 1 teaspoon dried thyme
- Salt and pepper to taste

INSTRUCTIONS:

1. Preheat oven to 400 degrees F (200 degrees C) and line a baking sheet with parchment paper.

2. In a large bowl, mix the delicata squash with the olive oil, thyme, salt, and pepper until equally covered.

3. Spread the delicata squash in a single layer on the prepared baking sheet.

4. Roast for 20 minutes, or until the delicata squash is soft and slightly caramelized.

5. Serve immediately.

Tips:

- For more savory side dish, add a sprinkling of grated Parmesan cheese or chopped fresh herbs before serving.

- To make the delicata squash extra crispy, roast it for an additional 5-10 minutes.

- For a deeper meal, sprinkle the delicata squash with a spoonful of honey or maple syrup before roasting.

ROASTED ASPARAGUS AND RED PEPPERS

- **Prep Time: 15 minutes**
- **Cooking Time: 20 minutes**
- **Serving Time: 5 minutes**

NUTRITIONAL VALUE (PER SERVING):

- Calories: 100
- Fat: 5g
- Saturated Fat: 0g
- Carbohydrates: 15g
- Fiber: 3g
- Sugar: 5g
- Protein: 3g

INGREDIENTS:

- 1-pound asparagus, trimmed
- 1 red bell pepper, sliced 1 tablespoon olive oil
- Salt and pepper to taste

INSTRUCTIONS:

1. Preheat oven to 400 degrees F (200 degrees C) and line a baking sheet with parchment paper.
2. In a large bowl, mix the asparagus and red pepper slices with the olive oil, salt, and pepper until equally coated.
3. Spread the asparagus and red pepper slices in a single layer on the prepared baking sheet.
4. Roast for 20 minutes, or until the asparagus is tender and slightly caramelized and the red peppers are softened.
5. Serve immediately.

Tips:

- For more savory side dish, add a sprinkle of grated Parmesan cheese or chopped fresh parsley before serving.
- To make the asparagus and red peppers extremely crispy, roast them for an additional 5-10 minutes.
- For a richer meal, sprinkle the asparagus and red peppers with a tablespoon of balsamic vinegar or honey before roasting.

TARRAGON SPRING PEAS

- **Prep Time: 5 minutes**
- **Cooking Time: 5 minutes**
- **Serving Time: 5 minutes**

NUTRITIONAL VALUE (PER SERVING):

- Calories: 100
- Fat: 3g
- Saturated Fat: 0g
- Carbohydrates: 15g
- Fiber: 2g
- Sugar: 2g
- Protein: 4g

INGREDIENTS:

- 1-pound fresh spring peas
- 1 tablespoon olive oil
- 1 teaspoon minced shallots
- 1/4 teaspoon dried tarragon
- Salt and pepper to taste

INSTRUCTIONS:

1. Bring a big saucepan of salted water to a boil.
2. Add the peas and simmer for 2-3 minutes, or until tender-crisp.
3. Drain the peas and leave aside.
4. In a large skillet, heat the olive oil over medium heat.
5. Add the shallots and sauté for 1 minute, or until softened.
6. Add the tarragon and simmer for 30 seconds, or until aromatic.
7. Add the peas and simmer for 1 minute, or until cooked through.
8. Season with salt and pepper to taste.
9. Serve immediately.

Tips:

- For more savory side dish, add a tablespoon of grated Parmesan cheese or a dollop of sour cream before serving.
- To make the peas more vivid, add a dash of lemon juice before serving.
- For a fuller meal, use fresh tarragon instead of dry tarragon.

Reciepe Card

COURSE: DIET: PREP TIME: COOK TIME: SERVINGS

INGREDIENTS

INSTRUCTIONS

Serves   Prep   Cook Time

TIPS & TRICKS

NOTES

SWEET POTATO AND ROASTED BEET SALAD

- **Prep Time: 15 minutes**
- **Cooking Time: 30 minutes**
- **Serving Time: 10 minutes**

NUTRITIONAL VALUE (PER SERVING):

- Calories: 400
- Fat: 15g
- Saturated Fat: 3g
- Carbohydrates: 50g
- Fiber: 10g
- Sugar: 20g
- Protein: 10g

INGREDIENTS:

- 1-pound sweet potato, peeled and sliced into 1-inch chunks
- 1 red beet, peeled and sliced into 1-inch chunks
- 2 tablespoons olive oil
- 1 tablespoon balsamic vinegar
- 1/2 teaspoon salt
- 1/4 teaspoon black pepper
- 1/4 cup chopped fresh parsley

INSTRUCTIONS:

1. Preheat oven to 400 degrees F (200 degrees C) and line a baking sheet with parchment paper.
2. In a large bowl, mix the sweet potato and beet cubes with the olive oil, balsamic vinegar, salt, and pepper until equally coated.
3. Spread the sweet potato and beet cubes in a single layer on the prepared baking sheet.
4. Roast for 30 minutes, or until the veggies are soft and slightly caramelized.
5. Let cool somewhat, then whisk in the parsley.
6. Serve immediately.

Tips:

- For more savory salad, add a sprinkle of chopped fresh cilantro or chives before serving.
- To make the salad extra crispy, bake the sweet potato and beet cubes for an additional 5-10 minutes.
- For a richer meal, add a spoonful of honey or maple syrup to the salad before serving.

HARVEST SALAD

- **Prep Time: 15 minutes**
- **Cooking Time: 0 minutes**
- **Serving Time: 5 minutes**

NUTRITIONAL VALUE (PER SERVING):

- Calories: 300
- Fat: 10g
- Saturated Fat: 2g
- Carbohydrates: 30g
- Fiber: 5g
- Sugar: 10g
- Protein: 15g

INGREDIENTS:

- 1 pound mixed greens
- 1/2 cup cooked quinoa
- 1/2 cup roasted butternut squash cubes
- 1/2 cup chopped apples
- 1/4 cup chopped walnuts
- 1/4 cup dried cranberries
- 2 teaspoons apple cider vinegar
- 1 tablespoon olive oil
- 1 teaspoon maple syrup
- 1/2 teaspoon salt
- 1/4 teaspoon black pepper

INSTRUCTIONS:

1. In a large bowl, combine the mixed greens, quinoa, butternut squash, apples, walnuts, and cranberries.
2. In a small bowl, mix together the apple cider vinegar, olive oil, maple syrup, salt, and pepper.
3. Drizzle the dressing over the salad and toss to coat.
4. Serve immediately.

Tips:

- For a more delicious salad, add a sprinkling of chopped fresh herbs, such as parsley, chives, or oregano, before serving.
- To make the salad extra crispy, add a handful of chopped romaine leaves before serving.
- For a richer meal, add a dollop of Greek yogurt or a spoonful of honey to the salad before serving.

ASIAN NOODLE SALAD

- **Prep Time: 15 minutes**
- **Cooking Time: 5 minutes**
- **Serving Time: 5 minutes**

NUTRITIONAL VALUE (PER SERVING):

- Calories: 350
- Fat: 12g
- Saturated Fat: 2g
- Carbohydrates: 45g
- Fiber: 3g
- Sugar: 5g
- Protein: 10g

INGREDIENTS:

- 8 ounces' rice noodles

- 2 teaspoons soy sauce
- 1 tablespoon rice vinegar
- 1 tablespoon sesame oil
- 1 teaspoon sriracha sauce
- 1/2 teaspoon ginger, grated
- 1/4 cup chopped peanuts
- 2 teaspoons chopped cilantro
- 2 green onions, finely sliced 1 carrot, shredded
- 1/2 cup red cabbage, shredded

INSTRUCTIONS:

1. Cook the rice noodles according per package guidelines.
2. Drain and rinse the noodles under cold water.
3. In a large bowl, mix together the soy sauce, rice vinegar, sesame oil, sriracha sauce, and ginger.
4. Add the noodles, peanuts, cilantro, green onions, carrot, and red cabbage to the bowl.
5. Toss to coat.
6. Serve immediately.

Tips:

- For a more delicious salad, marinate the noodles in the dressing for 30 minutes before serving.
- To make the salad extra crispy, add a handful of chopped romaine leaves before serving.
- For a richer meal, add a dollop of Greek yogurt or a spoonful of honey to the salad before serving.

HEALTHY TACO SALAD

- **Prep Time: 15 minutes**
- **Cooking Time: 15 minutes**
- **Serving Time: 5 minutes**

NUTRITIONAL VALUE (PER SERVING):

- Calories: 400
- Fat: 20g
- Saturated Fat: 5g
- Carbohydrates: 30g
- Fiber: 10g
- Sugar: 5g
- Protein: 30g

INGREDIENTS:

- 1-pound ground turkey or chicken, browned
- 1/2 teaspoon chili powder
- 1/4 teaspoon cumin
- 1/4 teaspoon salt
- 1/4 teaspoon black pepper
- 2 cups mixed greens
- 1 cup chopped tomatoes
- 1/2 cup chopped cucumber
- 1/4 cup chopped red onion 1/4 cup chopped avocado

- 2 tablespoons sour cream
- 1 tablespoon salsa
- 1 tablespoon chopped fresh cilantro

INSTRUCTIONS:

1. In a large pan, sauté the ground turkey or chicken over medium heat until browned.
2. Drain off any excess oil.
3. Season with the chili powder, cumin, salt, and pepper.
4. In a large bowl, combine the mixed greens, tomatoes, cucumber, red onion, avocado, sour cream, salsa, and cilantro.
5. Top with the cooked chicken.
6. Serve immediately.

CHICKEN GUACAMOLE SALAD

- **Prep Time: 10 minutes**
- **Cooking Time: 20 minutes**
- **Serving Time: 5 minutes**

NUTRITIONAL VALUE (PER SERVING):

- Calories: 350
- Fat: 15g
- Saturated Fat: 4g
- Carbohydrates: 20g
- Fiber: 5g
- Sugar: 2g
- Protein: 25g

INGREDIENTS:

- 2 cups cooked shredded chicken
- 1 ripe avocado, mashed
- 1/2 cup chopped red onion
- 1/4 cup chopped cilantro
- 2 teaspoons lime juice
- 1 tablespoon olive oil
- Salt and pepper to taste

INSTRUCTIONS:

1. In a large bowl, mix the cooked chicken, mashed avocado, red onion, cilantro, lime juice, and olive oil.
2. Season with salt and pepper to taste.
3. Serve immediately or refrigerate for later.

Tips:

- For more savory salad, add a touch of cayenne pepper or a splash of hot sauce.
- To make the salad extra creamy, add a spoonful of sour cream or Greek yogurt to the chicken mixture.
- For a more festive look, put the salad atop lettuce cups or in avocado halves.

WARM PORTOBELLO SALAD

- **Prep Time: 15 minutes**

- 💿 **Cooking Time: 20 minutes**
- 💿 **Serving Time: 5 minutes**

NUTRITIONAL VALUE (PER SERVING):

- 💿 Calories: 300
- 💿 Fat: 10g
- 💿 Saturated Fat: 2g
- 💿 Carbohydrates: 30g
- 💿 Fiber: 5g
- 💿 Sugar: 10g
- 💿 Protein: 15g

INGREDIENTS:

- 💿 2 Portobello mushroom tops, sliced
- 💿 1 tablespoon olive oil
- 💿 Salt and pepper to taste
- 💿 1/2 cup cooked quinoa
- 💿 1/4 cup chopped roasted red peppers
- 💿 1/4 cup chopped spinach
- 💿 2 tablespoons balsamic vinegar
- 💿 1 tablespoon olive oil
- 💿 1/4 teaspoon dried oregano
- 💿 Salt and pepper to taste

INSTRUCTIONS:

1. Preheat oven to 400 degrees F (200 degrees C).
2. In a large bowl, mix the Portobello mushroom slices with the olive oil, salt, and pepper.
3. Spread the mushroom slices in a single layer on a baking sheet.
4. Roast for 20 minutes, or until the mushrooms are soft.
5. In a small bowl, mix together the balsamic vinegar, olive oil, and oregano.
6. In a large bowl, mix the cooked quinoa, roasted red peppers, spinach, and balsamic dressing.
7. Top with the roasted Portobello mushroom slices.
8. Serve immediately.

Tips:

- For more savory salad, add a sprinkling of chopped fresh parsley or chives before serving.
- To make the salad extra crispy, bake the Portobello mushroom slices for an additional 5-10 minutes.
- For a richer meal, add a dollop of sour cream or Greek yogurt to the salad before serving.

LAYERED SALAD

- 💿 **Prep Time: 15 minutes**
- 💿 **Cooking Time: 0 minutes**
- 💿 **Serving Time: 5 minutes**

NUTRITIONAL VALUE (PER SERVING):

- 💿 Calories: 250

- Fat: 12g
- Saturated Fat: 2g
- Carbohydrates: 15g
- Fiber: 3g
- Sugar: 5g
- Protein: 5g

INGREDIENTS:

- 2 cups mixed greens
- 1/2 cup cherry tomatoes, halved
- 1/2 cup cucumber, sliced
- 1/4 cup red onion, thinly sliced
- 1/4 cup chopped fresh parsley
- 2 tablespoons olive oil
- 1 tablespoon balsamic vinegar
- 1/2 teaspoon salt
- 1/4 teaspoon black pepper

INSTRUCTIONS:

1. In a large bowl, add the mixed greens, cherry tomatoes, cucumber, red onion, and parsley.
2. In a small bowl, mix together the olive oil, balsamic vinegar, salt, and pepper.
3. Drizzle the dressing over the salad and toss to coat.
4. Serve immediately.

Tips:

- For more savory salad, add a sprinkling of chopped fresh herbs, such as basil, oregano, or thyme, before serving.
- To make the salad extra crispy, add a handful of chopped romaine leaves before serving.
- For a richer meal, add a dollop of sour cream or Greek yogurt to the salad before serving.

BAKED "POTATO" SALAD

- **Prep Time: 15 minutes**
- **Cooking Time: 45 minutes**
- **Serving Time: 5 minutes**

NUTRITIONAL VALUE (PER SERVING):

- Calories: 300
- Fat: 10g
- Saturated Fat: 2g
- Carbohydrates: 35g
- Fiber: 5g
- Sugar: 5g
- Protein: 15g

INGREDIENTS:

- 2 pounds' russet potatoes, peeled and cut into 1-inch chunks
- 2 tablespoons olive oil
- 1/2 teaspoon salt
- 1/4 teaspoon black pepper
- 1/4 cup mild sour cream
- 2 tablespoons chopped red onion
- 2 tablespoons chopped celery

2 teaspoons chopped fresh parsley

INSTRUCTIONS:

1. Preheat oven to 400 degrees F (200 degrees C).

2. In a large basin, mix the potatoes with the olive oil, salt, and pepper.

3. Spread the potatoes in a single layer on a baking sheet.

4. Bake for 45 minutes, or until the potatoes are soft and slightly browned.

5. Let cool slightly, then add the sour cream, red onion, celery, and parsley.

6. Mix gently to blend.

7. Serve immediately or refrigerate for later.

Tips:

- For more savory salad, add a sprinkle of chopped fresh chives or a touch of cayenne pepper before serving.

- To make the salad extra creamy, add a spoonful of Greek yogurt to the sour cream before adding to the potatoes.

- For a richer meal, add a spoonful of honey or maple syrup to the salad before serving.

CAPRESE SALAD

- **Prep Time: 10 minutes**
- **Cooking Time: 0 minutes**
- **Serving Time: 5 minutes**

NUTRITIONAL VALUE (PER SERVING):

- Calories: 200
- Fat: 12g
- Saturated Fat: 3g
- Carbohydrates: 10g
- Fiber: 2g
- Sugar: 3g
- Protein: 10g

INGREDIENTS:

- 1-pound cherry tomatoes, halved
- 1 ball of mozzarella cheese, sliced into bite-sized portions
- 12 fresh basil leaves
- 2 tablespoons olive oil
- 1 tablespoon balsamic vinegar
- Salt and pepper to taste

INSTRUCTIONS:

1. In a large bowl, mix the cherry tomatoes, mozzarella cheese, and basil leaves.

2. In a small bowl, mix together the olive oil, balsamic vinegar, salt, and pepper.

3. Drizzle the dressing over the salad and toss to coat.

4. Serve immediately.

Tips:

- For a more colorful meal, add a splash of lemon juice or red wine vinegar before serving.
- To add extra nutrition, garnish the salad with a sprinkling of chopped fresh parsley or oregano.
- For a richer meal, add a dollop of sour cream or Greek yogurt before serving.

ASIAN CUCUMBER SALAD

- **Prep Time: 10 minutes**
- **Cooking Time: 0 minutes**
- **Serving Time: 5 minutes**

NUTRITIONAL VALUE (PER SERVING):

- Calories: 50
- Fat: 2g
- Saturated Fat: 0g
- Carbohydrates: 5g
- Fiber: 2g
- Sugar: 2g
- Protein: 2g

INGREDIENTS:

- 2 cucumbers, sliced
- 1/4 cup rice vinegar
- 2 teaspoons soy sauce
- 1 tablespoon sesame oil
- 1 teaspoon ginger, grated
- 1/4 cup chopped fresh cilantro
- 1 tablespoon sesame seeds

INSTRUCTIONS:

1. In a large bowl, mix the cucumbers, rice vinegar, soy sauce, sesame oil, ginger, and cilantro.
2. Toss to coat.
3. Sprinkle with sesame seeds.
4. Serve immediately or refrigerate for later.

Tips:

- For more savory salad, add a sprinkle of red pepper flakes or a splash of hot sauce before serving.
- To make the salad extra crunchy, add a handful of chopped romaine lettuce or shredded cabbage before serving.
- For a richer meal, add a spoonful of honey or maple syrup to the dressing before adding to the cucumbers.

SCALLOP CAESAR SALAD

- **Prep Time: 15 minutes**
- **Cooking Time: 15 minutes**
- **Serving Time: 5 minutes**

NUTRITIONAL VALUE (PER SERVING):

- Calories: 400
- Fat: 25g

- Saturated Fat: 5g
- Carbohydrates: 10g
- Fiber: 2g
- Sugar: 2g
- Protein: 30g

INGREDIENTS:

- 1 pound scallops, patted dry
- 1 tablespoon olive oil
- Salt and pepper to taste
- 2 cups mixed greens
- 1/2 cup grated Parmesan cheese
- 1/4 cup croutons
- 2 tablespoons Caesar dressing

INSTRUCTIONS:

1. In a large pan, heat the olive oil over medium-high heat.
2. Season the scallops with salt and pepper.
3. Cook for 2-3 minutes each side, or until golden brown and heated through.
4. In a large bowl, combine the mixed greens, Parmesan cheese, croutons, and Caesar dressing.
5. Top with the cooked scallops.
6. Serve immediately.

Tips:

- For a more delicious salad, add a sprinkling of chopped fresh anchovies or a dash of cayenne pepper before serving.
- To make the salad extra crunchy, add a handful of chopped romaine lettuce or a sprinkling of sunflower seeds before serving.
- For a richer meal, add a dollop of sour cream or Greek yogurt to the Caesar dressing before adding to the salad.

CHICKEN SALAD IN CUCUMBER CUPS

- **Prep Time: 20 minutes**
- **Cooking Time: 15 minutes**
- **Serving Time: 10 minutes**

NUTRITIONAL VALUE (PER SERVING):

- Calories: 350
- Fat: 15g
- Saturated Fat: 4g
- Carbohydrates: 15g
- Fiber: 3g
- Sugar: 2g
- Protein: 25g

INGREDIENTS:

- 2 cups cooked shredded chicken
- 1/4 cup chopped celery 1/4 cup chopped red onion
- 2 teaspoons chopped green onion

- 2 tablespoons mayonnaise
- 1 tablespoon lemon juice
- Salt and pepper to taste
- 4 cucumbers, halved and hollowed out

INSTRUCTIONS:

1. In a large bowl, add the cooked chicken, celery, red onion, green onion, mayonnaise, lemon juice, salt, and pepper.
2. Mix gently to blend.
3. Spoon the chicken salad into the cucumber cups.
4. Serve immediately or refrigerate for later.

Tips:

- For more savory salad, add a sprinkling of chopped fresh herbs, such as parsley, tarragon, or dill, before serving.
- To make the salad extra crunchy, add a handful of chopped iceberg lettuce or a sprinkling of chopped almonds before serving.
- For a richer meal, add a dollop of sour cream or Greek yogurt to the chicken salad before serving.

SUNFLOWER SEEDS AND ARUGULA GARDEN SALAD

- **Prep Time: 10 minutes**
- **Cooking Time: 0 minutes**
- **Serving Time: 5 minutes**

NUTRITIONAL VALUE (PER SERVING):

- Calories: 100
- Fat: 6g
- Saturated Fat: 1g
- Carbohydrates: 5g
- Fiber: 2g
- Sugar: 3g
- Protein: 3g

INGREDIENTS:

- 2 cups arugula
- 1/4 cup sunflower seeds
- 1/4 cup cherry tomatoes, halved
- 2 tablespoons olive oil
- 1 tablespoon lemon juice
- Salt and pepper to taste

INSTRUCTIONS:

1. In a large bowl, mix the arugula, sunflower seeds, and cherry tomatoes.
2. In a small bowl, mix together the olive oil, lemon juice, salt, and pepper.
3. Drizzle the dressing over the salad and toss to coat.
4. Serve immediately.

- For more savory salad, add a sprinkling of chopped fresh herbs, such as parsley, basil, or oregano, before serving.
- To make the salad extra crunchy, add a handful of chopped romaine lettuce or a sprinkling of chopped nuts before serving.
- For a richer meal, add a dollop of sour cream or Greek yogurt to the dressing before adding to the salad.

SUPREME CAESAR SALAD

- **Prep Time: 15 minutes**
- **Cooking Time: 20 minutes**
- **Serving Time: 5 minutes**

NUTRITIONAL VALUE (PER SERVING):

- Calories: 450
- Fat: 28g
- Saturated Fat: 7g
- Carbohydrates: 15g
- Fiber: 4g
- Sugar: 3g
- Protein: 35g

INGREDIENTS:

- 1-pound rotisserie chicken, skin removed and shredded
- 2 cups romaine lettuce, chopped
- 1/2 cup grated Parmesan cheese
- 1/4 cup croutons
- 2 tablespoons Caesar dressing

INSTRUCTIONS:

1. In a large bowl, mix the rotisserie chicken, romaine lettuce, Parmesan cheese, croutons, and Caesar dressing.
2. Toss to coat.
3. Top with extra Parmesan cheese, if preferred.
4. Serve immediately.

Tips:

- For a more delicious salad, add a sprinkling of chopped fresh anchovies or a dash of cayenne pepper before serving.
- To make the salad extra crunchy, add a handful of chopped romaine lettuce or a sprinkling of sunflower seeds before serving.
- For a richer meal, add a dollop of sour cream or Greek yogurt to the Caesar dressing before adding to the salad.

DILL CELERY SOUP

- **Prep Time: 10 minutes**
- **Cooking Time: 20 minutes**
- **Serving Time: 5 minutes**

NUTRITIONAL VALUE (PER SERVING):

- Calories: 75
- Fat: 3g
- Saturated Fat: 1g
- Carbohydrates: 10g
- Fiber: 2g
- Sugar: 2g
- Protein: 3g

INGREDIENTS:

- 2 tablespoons olive oil
- 1 onion, chopped 2 celery stalks, chopped 2 cups vegetable broth
- 1/2 cup chopped fresh dill
- Salt and pepper to taste

INSTRUCTIONS:

1. In a large saucepan, heat the olive oil over medium heat.
2. Add the onion and celery and simmer until softened, approximately 5 minutes.
3. Stir in the veggie broth and dill.
4. Bring to a boil, then decrease heat and simmer for 15 minutes, or until the celery is soft.
5. Season with salt and pepper to taste.
6. Serve immediately.

Tips:

- For a smoother soup, purée it in a blender before serving.
- To make the soup tastier, add a bit of cayenne pepper or a splash of lemon juice before serving.
- For a richer meal, add a dollop of sour cream or Greek yogurt before serving.

CREAMY AVOCADO-BROCCOLI SOUP

- **Prep Time: 15 minutes**
- **Cooking Time: 25 minutes**
- **Serving Time: 5 minutes**

NUTRITIONAL VALUE (PER SERVING):

- Calories: 200
- Fat: 12g
- Saturated Fat: 2g
- Carbohydrates: 15g
- Fiber: 4g
- Sugar: 5g
- Protein: 5g

INGREDIENTS:

- 1 tablespoon olive oil
- 1 onion, chopped
- 2 cloves garlic, minced
- 1 head of broccoli, florets only
- 2 cups vegetable broth 1/2 ripe avocado, mashed
- 1/4 cup low-fat milk or Greek yogurt
- Salt and pepper to taste

INSTRUCTIONS:

1. In a large saucepan, heat the olive oil over medium heat.
2. Add the onion and simmer until softened, approximately 5 minutes.
3. Add the garlic and simmer for 1 minute longer.
4. Stir in the broccoli and vegetable broth.
5. Bring to a boil, then decrease heat and simmer for 15 minutes, or until the broccoli is soft.
6. Remove from heat and let cool slightly.
7. Stir in the mashed avocado, milk or yogurt, salt, and pepper.
8. Blend the soup till smooth.
9. Serve immediately.

Tips:

- For a more delicious soup, add a bit of cayenne pepper or a splash of lemon juice before serving.
- To make the soup extra creamy, add an additional tablespoon of milk or yogurt before serving.
- For a richer meal, add a dollop of sour cream or Greek yogurt before serving.

FRESH GARDEN VEGETABLE SOUP

- **Prep Time: 15 minutes**
- **Cooking Time: 30 minutes**
- **Serving Time: 5 minutes**

NUTRITIONAL VALUE (PER SERVING):

- Calories: 125
- Fat: 4g
- Saturated Fat: 1g
- Carbohydrates: 20g
- Fiber: 5g
- Sugar: 5g
- Protein: 4g

INGREDIENTS:

- 2 tablespoons olive oil
- 1 onion, chopped 2 carrots, chopped 2 celery stalks, chopped 2 cups vegetable broth

1 (14.5-ounce) can diced tomatoes, undrained 1 cup chopped fresh spinach

Salt and pepper to taste

INSTRUCTIONS:

1. In a large saucepan, heat the olive oil over medium heat.
2. Add the onion, carrots, and celery and simmer until softened, approximately 5 minutes.
3. Stir in the veggie broth, chopped tomatoes, and spinach.
4. Bring to a boil, then decrease heat and simmer for 15 minutes, or until the veggies are soft.
5. Season with salt and pepper to taste.
6. Serve immediately.

Tips:

- For more savory soup, add a sprinkle of dried thyme or oregano before serving.
- To make the soup more substantial, add a cooked and diced chicken breast before serving.
- For a richer meal, add a dollop of sour cream or Greek yogurt before serving.

SWISS CAULIFLOWER-EMMENTAL-SOUP

Prep Time: 10 minutes

Cooking Time: 20 minutes

Serving Time: 5 minutes

NUTRITIONAL VALUE (PER SERVING):

Calories: 150

Fat: 10g

Saturated Fat: 6g

Carbohydrates: 10g

Fiber: 2g

Sugar: 2g

Protein: 7g

INGREDIENTS:

1 tablespoon olive oil

1 onion, chopped

1 head of cauliflower, florets only

2 cups vegetable broth

1/2 cup shredded Swiss cheese

1/4 cup grated Parmesan cheese

Salt and pepper to taste

INSTRUCTIONS:

1. In a large saucepan, heat the olive oil over medium heat.
2. Add the onion and simmer until softened, approximately 5 minutes.
3. Stir in the cauliflower and vegetable broth.
4. Bring to a boil, then decrease heat and simmer for 15 minutes, or until the cauliflower is soft.

5. Remove from heat and toss in the Swiss cheese, Parmesan cheese, salt, and pepper.

6. Let cool slightly, then mix the soup until smooth.

7. Serve immediately.

Tips:

- For a more flavored soup, add a touch of nutmeg or a splash of lemon juice before serving.

- To make the soup extra creamy, add an additional tablespoon of olive oil or a dollop of sour cream before serving.

- For a richer meal, add a dollop of sour cream or Greek yogurt before serving.

CHILLED AVOCADO TOMATO SOUP

- **Prep Time: 15 minutes**
- **Cooking Time: 0 minutes**
- **Serving Time: 10 minutes**
- **Total Time: 25 minutes**

NUTRITIONAL VALUE (PER SERVING):

- Calories: 250
- Fat: 15g
- Saturated Fat: 2g
- Carbohydrates: 15g
- Fiber: 3g
- Sugar: 5g
- Protein: 5g

INGREDIENTS:

- 1 ripe avocado, mashed 1 (14.5-ounce) can chopped tomatoes, undrained
- 1/2 cup vegetable broth 1/4 cup chopped red onion
- 1/4 cup chopped fresh cilantro
- 1 tablespoon lime juice
- Salt and pepper to taste

INSTRUCTIONS:

1. In a large bowl, mix the mashed avocado, diced tomatoes, vegetable broth, red onion, cilantro, lime juice, salt, and pepper.

2. Mix thoroughly until smooth.

3. Cover and refrigerate in the refrigerator for at least 1 hour, or up to overnight.

4. Serve cold.

Tips:

- For a more delicious soup, add a bit of cayenne pepper or a splash of hot sauce before serving.

- To make the soup extra creamy, add one additional tablespoon of vegetable stock or a dollop of sour cream before serving.

- For a richer meal, add a dollop of sour cream or Greek yogurt before serving.

PUMPKIN AND WHITE BEAN SOUP WITH SAGE

- **Prep Time: 15 minutes**
- **Cooking Time: 30 minutes**
- **Serving Time: 5 minutes**
- **Total Time: 50 minutes**

NUTRITIONAL VALUE (PER SERVING):

- Calories: 200
- Fat: 8g
- Saturated Fat: 1g
- Carbohydrates: 30g
- Fiber: 6g
- Sugar: 4g
- Protein: 8g

INGREDIENTS:

- 1 tablespoon olive oil
- 1 onion, chopped
- 2 cloves garlic, minced
- 1 (15-ounce) can pumpkin puree
- 1 (15-ounce) can cannellini beans, drained and rinsed
- 4 cups vegetable broth
- 1 teaspoon dried sage
- Salt and pepper to taste

INSTRUCTIONS:

1. In a large saucepan, heat the olive oil over medium heat.
2. Add the onion and simmer until softened, approximately 5 minutes.
3. Add the garlic and simmer for 1 minute longer.
4. Stir in the pumpkin puree, cannellini beans, vegetable broth, sage, salt, and pepper.
5. Bring to a boil, then decrease heat and simmer for 20 minutes, or until the soup is cooked through.
6. Serve immediately.

Tips:

- For a more flavored soup, add a touch of nutmeg or a dash of cinnamon before serving.
- To make the soup extra creamy, add an additional tablespoon of olive oil or a dollop of sour cream before serving.
- For a richer meal, add a dollop of sour cream or Greek yogurt before serving.

ALKALINE CARROT SOUP WITH MILLET

- **Prep Time: 20 minutes**
- **Cooking Time: 40 minutes**
- **Serving Time: 5 minutes**
- **Total Time: 65 minutes**

NUTRITIONAL VALUE (PER SERVING):

- Calories: 225
- Fat: 8g
- Saturated Fat: 2g
- Carbohydrates: 35g
- Fiber: 6g
- Sugar: 5g
- Protein: 6g

INGREDIENTS:

- 2 tablespoons olive oil
- 1 onion, chopped 2 cloves garlic, minced 1 pound carrots, peeled and chopped 1/2 cup millet, washed
- 4 cups vegetable broth
- 1/4 cup chopped fresh parsley
- Salt and pepper to taste

INSTRUCTIONS:

1. In a large saucepan, heat the olive oil over medium heat.
2. Add the onion and simmer until softened, approximately 5 minutes.
3. Add the garlic and simmer for 1 minute longer.
4. Stir in the carrots and millet.
5. Cook for 5 minutes, stirring periodically.
6. Stir in the veggie broth and bring to a boil.
7. Reduce heat and simmer for 30 minutes, or until the carrots and millet are soft.
8. Stir in the parsley, salt, and pepper.
9. Serve immediately.

ALKALINE PUMPKIN TOMATO SOUP

- **Prep Time: 15 minutes**
- **Cooking Time: 20 minutes**
- **Serving Time: 5 minutes**
- **Total Time: 40 minutes**

NUTRITIONAL VALUE (PER SERVING):

- Calories: 175
- Fat: 7g
- Saturated Fat: 1g
- Carbohydrates: 25g
- Fiber: 5g
- Sugar: 4g
- Protein: 4g

INGREDIENTS:

- 2 tablespoons olive oil
- 1 onion, chopped
- 2 cloves garlic, minced
- 1 (15-ounce) can pumpkin puree
- 1 (14.5-ounce) can chopped tomatoes, undrained
- 4 cups vegetable broth
- 1/4 cup chopped fresh basil
- Salt and pepper to taste

INSTRUCTIONS:

1. In a large saucepan, heat the olive oil over medium heat.

2. Add the onion and simmer until softened, approximately 5 minutes.

3. Add the garlic and simmer for 1 minute longer.

4. Stir in the pumpkin puree, diced tomatoes, vegetable broth, and basil.

5. Bring to a boil, then decrease heat and simmer for 15 minutes, or until the soup is cooked through.

6. Season with salt and pepper to taste.

7. Serve immediately.

Tips:

- For a more colorful soup, add a drop of red wine vinegar before serving.

- To make the soup extra creamy, add an additional tablespoon of olive oil or a dollop of sour cream before serving.

- For a richer meal, add a dollop of sour cream or Greek yogurt before serving.

COLD CAULIFLOWER-COCONUT SOUP

- **Prep Time: 10 minutes**
- **Cooking Time: 20 minutes**
- **Serving Time: 1 hour**
- **Total Time: 1 hour 30 minutes**

NUTRITIONAL VALUE (PER SERVING):

- Calories: 150
- Fat: 10g
- Saturated Fat: 6g
- Carbohydrates: 10g
- Fiber: 3g
- Sugar: 3g
- Protein: 3g

INGREDIENTS:

- 1 head of cauliflower, florets only
- 1 (14-ounce) can low-fat coconut milk
- 1/4 cup chopped fresh cilantro
- 1 tablespoon lime juice
- Salt and pepper to taste

INSTRUCTIONS:

1. In a large saucepan, mix the cauliflower florets, coconut milk, cilantro, lime juice, salt, and pepper.

2. Bring to a boil, then decrease heat and simmer for 15 minutes, or until the cauliflower is soft.

3. Remove from heat and let cool slightly.

4. Using an immersion blender or normal blender, mix the soup until smooth.

5. Pour the soup into a bowl and cover with plastic wrap.

6. Refrigerate for at least 1 hour, or up to overnight.

7. Serve cold.

- For a more flavored soup, add a touch of curry powder or a splash of turmeric before serving.

- To make the soup extra creamy, add an additional tablespoon of coconut milk before serving.

- For a richer meal, add a dollop of sour cream or Greek yogurt before serving.

RAW AVOCADO-BROCCOLI SOUP WITH CASHEW NUTS

- **Prep Time: 15 minutes**
- **Cooking Time: 0 minutes**
- **Serving Time: 5 minutes**
- **Total Time: 20 minutes**

NUTRITIONAL VALUE (PER SERVING):

- Calories: 300
- Fat: 18g
- Saturated Fat: 3g
- Carbohydrates: 15g
- Fiber: 4g
- Sugar: 5g
- Protein: 5g

INGREDIENTS:

- 1 ripe avocado, peeled and pitted
- 1 head of broccoli, florets only
- 1/2 cup raw cashews, soaking for 2 hours
- 1/4 cup chopped fresh parsley
- 1/4 cup water, or more as required
- Salt and pepper to taste

INSTRUCTIONS:

1. In a high-powered blender, add the avocado, broccoli, soaked cashews, parsley, and water.
2. Blend until smooth and creamy, adding additional water as required.
3. Season with salt and pepper to taste.
4. Serve immediately or refrigerate for later.

Tips:

- For a more flavored soup, add a touch of garlic powder or a dash of cayenne pepper before serving.

- To make the soup extra creamy, add an additional spoonful of soaked cashews before serving.

- For a richer meal, add a dollop of sour cream or Greek yogurt before serving.

KALE CAULIFLOWER SOUP

- **Prep Time: 15 minutes**
- **Cooking Time: 20 minutes**
- **Serving Time: 5 minutes**

- **Total Time: 40 minutes**

NUTRITIONAL VALUE (PER SERVING):

- Calories: 150
- Fat: 5g
- Saturated Fat: 1g
- Carbohydrates: 15g
- Fiber: 5g
- Sugar: 5g
- Protein: 4g

INGREDIENTS:

- 1 tablespoon olive oil
- 1 onion, chopped 2 cloves garlic, minced
- 1 head of cauliflower, florets only 1 bunch of kale, chopped 4 cups vegetable broth 1/4 cup chopped fresh parsley
- Salt and pepper to taste

INSTRUCTIONS:

1. In a large saucepan, heat the olive oil over medium heat.
2. Add the onion and simmer until softened, approximately 5 minutes.
3. Add the garlic and simmer for 1 minute longer.
4. Stir in the cauliflower and greens.
5. Cook for 5 minutes, stirring periodically.
6. Stir in the veggie broth, parsley, salt, and pepper.
7. Bring to a boil, then decrease heat and simmer for 15 minutes, or until the cauliflower and kale are soft.
8. Serve immediately.

Tips:

- For a more delicious soup, add a sprinkle of dried thyme or a dash of nutmeg before serving.
- To make the soup extra creamy, add an additional tablespoon of olive oil or a dollop of sour cream before serving.
- For a richer meal, add a dollop of sour cream or Greek yogurt before serving.

HEALTHY BROCCOLI ASPARAGUS SOUP

- **Prep Time: 10 minutes**
- **Cooking Time: 20 minutes**
- **Serving Time: 5 minutes**
- **Total Time: 35 minutes**

NUTRITIONAL VALUE (PER SERVING):

- Calories: 75
- Fat: 3g
- Saturated Fat: 1g
- Carbohydrates: 10g
- Fiber: 3g
- Sugar: 3g

- Protein: 4g

INGREDIENTS:

- 2 tablespoons olive oil
- 1 onion, chopped
- 2 cloves garlic, minced
- 2 cups broccoli florets
- 1 cup asparagus spears, trimmed and chopped
- 4 cups vegetable broth
- 1/4 cup chopped fresh parsley
- Salt and pepper to taste
- Optional garnishes: chopped fresh dill, lemon wedges

INSTRUCTIONS:

1. In a large saucepan, heat the olive oil over medium heat.
2. Add the onion and simmer until softened, approximately 5 minutes.
3. Add the garlic and simmer for 1 minute longer.
4. Stir in the broccoli and asparagus.
5. Cook for 5 minutes, stirring periodically.
6. Stir in the veggie broth, parsley, salt, and pepper.
7. Bring to a boil, then decrease heat and simmer for 15 minutes, or until the veggies are soft.
8. Serve immediately, topped with chopped fresh dill and lemon wedges, if preferred.

Tips:

- For a smoother soup, purée it in a blender before serving.
- To make the soup tastier, add a bit of cayenne pepper or a splash of lemon juice before serving.
- For a richer meal, add a dollop of sour cream or Greek yogurt before serving.

CREAMY ASPARAGUS SOUP

- **Prep Time: 15 minutes**
- **Cooking Time: 20 minutes**
- **Serving Time: 5 minutes**
- **Total Time: 40 minutes**

NUTRITIONAL VALUE (PER SERVING):

- Calories: 150
- Fat: 10g
- Saturated Fat: 6g
- Carbohydrates: 15g
- Fiber: 4g
- Sugar: 5g
- Protein: 4g

INGREDIENTS:

- 1 tablespoon olive oil

- 1 onion, chopped
- 2 cloves garlic, minced
- 2 cups asparagus spears, trimmed and chopped
- 1/2 cup thick cream
- 1/4 cup grated Parmesan cheese
- 4 cups vegetable broth
- Salt and pepper to taste
- Optional garnishes: chopped fresh chives, pieces of baguette

INSTRUCTIONS:

1. In a large saucepan, heat the olive oil over medium heat.
2. Add the onion and simmer until softened, approximately 5 minutes.
3. Add the garlic and simmer for 1 minute longer.
4. Stir in the asparagus and simmer for 5 minutes, stirring regularly.
5. In a blender, mix the heavy cream, Parmesan cheese, vegetable broth, salt, and pepper. Blend until smooth.
6. Pour the combined mixture into the saucepan with the asparagus and heat to a boil.
7. Reduce heat and simmer for 10 minutes, or until the asparagus is tender.
8. Serve immediately, topped with chopped fresh chives and slices of baguette, if preferred.

Tips:

- For a thicker soup, add an extra tablespoon of heavy cream before serving.
- For a healthy soup, add low-fat or dairy-free cream.
- For a spicy soup, add a sprinkle of red pepper flakes before serving.

TROUT BAKE

- **Prep Time: 10 minutes**
- **Cooking Time: 20 minutes**
- **Serving Time: 5 minutes**
- **Total Time: 35 minutes**

NUTRITIONAL VALUE (PER SERVING):

- Calories: 350
- Fat: 15g
- Saturated Fat: 5g
- Carbohydrates: 10g
- Fiber: 2g
- Sugar: 5g
- Protein: 30g

INGREDIENTS:

- 2 fish fillets, skin on 1 tablespoon olive oil
- 1/2 lemon, sliced
- 1 teaspoon dried thyme
- 1/4 teaspoon salt
- 1/4 teaspoon black pepper
- 1 cup chopped fresh veggies (such as carrots, celery, and onions)

INSTRUCTIONS:

1. Preheat oven to 375 degrees F (190 degrees C).
2. Line a baking pan with foil.
3. Place the fish fillets on the prepared baking sheet.
4. Drizzle the trout with olive oil.
5. Top the fish with lemon slices, thyme, salt, and pepper.
6. Arrange the chopped veggies around the trout.
7. Bake for 20 minutes, or until the fish is cooked through and the veggies are soft.
8. Serve immediately.

Tips:

- For a more delicious meal, add a touch of garlic powder or a dash of paprika before baking.
- To make the dish particularly moist, add a tablespoon of butter or margarine to the veggies before baking.
- For a richer meal, serve the fish with a dollop of sour cream or Greek yogurt.

SWORDFISH STEAK

- **Prep Time: 10 minutes**
- **Cooking Time: 15 minutes**
- **Serving Time: 5 minutes**
- **Total Time: 30 minutes**

- Calories: 300
- Fat: 12g
- Saturated Fat: 3g
- Carbohydrates: 0g
- Fiber: 0g
- Sugar: 0g
- Protein: 45g

INGREDIENTS:

- 2 swordfish steaks, approximately 1 inch thick
- 1 tablespoon olive oil
- 1/2 lemon, sliced
- 1 teaspoon dried oregano
- 1/4 teaspoon salt
- 1/4 teaspoon black pepper

INSTRUCTIONS:

1. Preheat grill or grill pan to medium-high heat.
2. Drizzle the swordfish steaks with olive oil.
3. Grill the swordfish steaks for 4-5 minutes each side, or until cooked through.
4. Transfer the swordfish steaks to a platter and cover with lemon slices, oregano, salt, and pepper.
5. Serve immediately.

Tips:

- For a more delicious dinner, marinate the swordfish steaks in your preferred marinade for at least 30 minutes before grilling.
- To make the meal extra juicy, baste the swordfish steaks with olive oil or butter while cooking.
- For a richer meal, serve the swordfish steaks with a dollop of sour cream or Greek yogurt.

SHRIMP COCONUT CURRY

- **Prep Time: 10 minutes**
- **Cooking Time: 20 minutes**
- **Serving Time: 5 minutes**
- **Total Time: 35 minutes**

NUTRITIONAL VALUE (PER SERVING):

- Calories: 250
- Fat: 14g
- Saturated Fat: 4g
- Carbohydrates: 15g
- Fiber: 5g
- Sugar: 10g
- Protein: 25g

INGREDIENTS:

- 1-pound shrimp, peeled and deveined
- 1 tablespoon olive oil
- 1 onion, chopped

- 2 cloves garlic, minced
- 1 tablespoon curry powder
- 1 (14-ounce) can coconut milk
- 1 cup vegetable broth
- 1/2 cup chopped fresh cilantro
- Salt and pepper to taste

INSTRUCTIONS:

1. Heat the olive oil in a large skillet or saucepan over medium heat.
2. Add the onion and simmer until softened, approximately 5 minutes.
3. Add the garlic and simmer for 1 minute longer.
4. Stir in the curry powder and simmer for 30 seconds, until aromatic.
5. Add the coconut milk, vegetable broth, shrimp, cilantro, salt, and pepper.
6. Bring to a boil, then decrease heat and simmer for 5-7 minutes, or until the shrimp is cooked through.
7. Serve immediately.

Tips:

- For a more delicious curry, add a touch of turmeric or a dash of ginger powder before cooking.
- To make the curry extra creamy, add an additional tablespoon of coconut milk before serving.
- For a healthy curry, use low-fat or dairy-free coconut milk.

TUNA AND CHEDDAR

- **Prep Time: 10 minutes**
- **Cooking Time: 15 minutes**
- **Serving Time: 5 minutes**
- **Total Time: 30 minutes**

NUTRITIONAL VALUE (PER SERVING):

- Calories: 400
- Fat: 20g
- Saturated Fat: 8g
- Carbohydrates: 10g
- Fiber: 2g
- Sugar: 5g
- Protein: 35g

INGREDIENTS:

- 2 cans (6 ounces each) tuna, drained and flakes
- 1 (8-ounce) can cream of mushroom soup
- 1/2 cup shredded cheddar cheese
- 1/4 cup chopped onion
- 1/4 cup chopped celery
- Salt and pepper to taste

INSTRUCTIONS:

1. Preheat oven to 350 degrees F (175 degrees C).
2. Grease a 9x13-inch baking dish.

3. In a medium bowl, mix the tuna, cream of mushroom soup, cheddar cheese, onion, celery, salt, and pepper.

4. Mix thoroughly.

5. Pour the mixture into the prepared baking dish.

6. Bake for 15 minutes, or until cooked through and bubbling.

7. Serve immediately.

Tips:

- For a more delicious meal, add a touch of garlic powder or a dash of paprika before baking.

- To make the dish extra creamy, add an additional tablespoon of milk before baking.

- For a richer dish, top the casserole with an extra 1/4 cup of shredded cheddar cheese before baking.

CHILI SHRIMP

- **Prep Time: 10 minutes**
- **Cooking Time: 15 minutes**
- **Serving Time: 5 minutes**
- **Total Time: 30 minutes**

NUTRITIONAL VALUE (PER SERVING):

- Calories: 200
- Fat: 10g
- Saturated Fat: 3g
- Carbohydrates: 15g
- Fiber: 3g
- Sugar: 5g
- Protein: 25g

INGREDIENTS:

- 1-pound shrimp, peeled and deveined
- 1 tablespoon olive oil
- 1 onion, chopped
- 2 cloves garlic, minced
- 1 tablespoon chili powder
- 1 (14-ounce) can chopped tomatoes, undrained
- 1/2 cup vegetable broth
- Salt and pepper to taste

INSTRUCTIONS:

1. Heat the olive oil in a large skillet or saucepan over medium heat.

2. Add the onion and simmer until softened, approximately 5 minutes.

3. Add the garlic and simmer for 1 minute longer.

4. Stir in the chili powder and simmer for 30 seconds, until aromatic.

5. Add the diced tomatoes, vegetable broth, shrimp, salt, and pepper.

6. Bring to a boil, then decrease heat and simmer for 5-7 minutes, or until the shrimp is cooked through.

7. Serve immediately.

Tips:

- For a more delicious chili, add a sprinkle of cumin or a dash of oregano before cooking.

- To make the chili extremely spicy, add a sprinkle of cayenne pepper before serving.

- For a richer chili, top the chili with a dollop of sour cream or Greek yogurt.

MUSSELS WITH SPAGHETTI SQUASH

- **Prep Time: 15 minutes**
- **Cooking Time: 20 minutes**
- **Serving Time: 5 minutes**
- **Total Time: 40 minutes**

NUTRITIONAL VALUE (PER SERVING):

- Calories: 250
- Fat: 12g
- Saturated Fat: 3g
- Carbohydrates: 20g
- Fiber: 5g
- Sugar: 5g
- Protein: 25g

INGREDIENTS:

- 1 pound mussels, washed and debearded
- 1 tablespoon olive oil
- 1 onion, chopped
- 2 cloves garlic, minced
- 1 (14-ounce) can chopped tomatoes, undrained
- 1/2 cup white wine
- 1/2 cup chopped fresh parsley
- Salt and pepper to taste
- 1 spaghetti squash, boiled and shredded

INSTRUCTIONS:

1. Heat the olive oil in a big saucepan over medium heat.
2. Add the onion and simmer until softened, approximately 5 minutes.
3. Add the garlic and simmer for 1 minute longer.
4. Stir in the diced tomatoes, white wine, parsley, salt, and pepper.
5. Bring to a boil, then decrease heat and simmer for 10 minutes.
6. Add the mussels and simmer, covered, until the mussels have opened, approximately 5-7 minutes.
7. Discard any mussels that do not open.
8. Serve the mussels over the shredded spaghetti squash.

Tips:

- For more savory meal, add a touch of red pepper flakes or a dash of cayenne pepper before cooking.

- To make the meal really garlicky, add an additional clove of garlic before cooking.
- For a richer meal, add a dollop of sour cream or Greek yogurt to the mussels before serving.

COD WITH WHITE SAUCE

- **Prep Time: 10 minutes**
- **Cooking Time: 15 minutes**
- **Serving Time: 5 minutes**
- **Total Time: 30 minutes**

NUTRITIONAL VALUE (PER SERVING):

- Calories: 350
- Fat: 15g
- Saturated Fat: 5g
- Carbohydrates: 10g
- Fiber: 2g
- Sugar: 5g
- Protein: 35g

INGREDIENTS:

- 1-pound cod fillets
- 1 tablespoon olive oil
- 1 onion, chopped
- 2 cloves garlic, minced
- 1/4 cup all-purpose flour
- 2 cups milk
- 1/4 cup grated Parmesan cheese
- Salt and pepper to taste

INSTRUCTIONS:

1. Preheat oven to 375 degrees F (190 degrees C).
2. Grease a 9x13-inch baking dish.
3. Pat the cod fillets dry with paper towels.
4. Season the fish fillets with salt and pepper.
5. Heat the olive oil in a large pan over medium heat.
6. Add the onion and simmer until softened, approximately 5 minutes.
7. Add the garlic and simmer for 1 minute longer.
8. Stir in the flour and cook for 1 minute, until golden brown.
9. Gradually whisk in the milk until smooth.
10. Bring to a boil, then decrease heat and simmer for 10 minutes, or until the sauce is thickened.
11. Stir in the Parmesan cheese.
12. Place the fish fillets in the prepared baking dish.
13. Pour the white sauce over the fish fillets.
14. Bake for 15 minutes, or until the fish is cooked through.
15. Serve immediately.

Tips:

- For more savory meal, add a touch of nutmeg or a dash of paprika before cooking.
- To make the dish extra creamy, add an additional tablespoon of milk before baking.
- For a richer meal, cover the fish with an extra 1/4 cup of grated Parmesan cheese before baking.

LEMON SOLE

- **Prep Time: 10 minutes**
- **Cooking Time: 15 minutes**
- **Serving Time: 5 minutes**
- **Total Time: 30 minutes**

NUTRITIONAL VALUE (PER SERVING):

- Calories: 300
- Fat: 12g
- Saturated Fat: 3g
- Carbohydrates: 0g
- Fiber: 0g
- Sugar: 0g
- Protein: 45g

INGREDIENTS:

- 2 lemon sole fillets
- 1 tablespoon olive oil
- 1/2 lemon, sliced
- 1 teaspoon dried thyme
- 1/4 teaspoon salt
- 1/4 teaspoon black pepper

INSTRUCTIONS:

1. Preheat grill or grill pan to medium-high heat.
2. Drizzle the lemon sole fillets with olive oil.
3. Grill the lemon sole fillets for 4-5 minutes each side, or until cooked through.
4. Transfer the lemon sole fillets to a platter and cover with lemon slices, thyme, salt, and pepper.
5. Serve immediately.

Tips:

- For a more delicious dinner, marinate the lemon sole fillets in your preferred marinade for at least 30 minutes before grilling.
- To make the meal extra juicy, baste the lemon sole fillets with olive oil or butter while cooking.
- For a richer meal, serve the lemon sole fillets with a dollop of sour cream or Greek yogurt.

COD IN PARSLEY SAUCE

- **Prep Time: 10 minutes**
- **Cooking Time: 15 minutes**

- **Serving Time: 5 minutes**
- **Total Time: 30 minutes**

NUTRITIONAL VALUE (PER SERVING):

- Calories: 250
- Fat: 10g
- Saturated Fat: 3g
- Carbohydrates: 5g
- Fiber: 1g
- Sugar: 2g
- Protein: 30g

INGREDIENTS:

- 2 cod fillets
- 1 tablespoon olive oil
- 1/4 cup chopped fresh parsley
- 1/4 cup lemon juice
- 2 cloves garlic, minced
- Salt and pepper to taste

INSTRUCTIONS:

1. Preheat grill or grill pan to medium-high heat.
2. Drizzle the cod fillets with olive oil.
3. Grill the fish fillets for 4-5 minutes each side, or until cooked through.
4. In a small bowl, mix the parsley, lemon juice, garlic, salt, and pepper.
5. Spoon the parsley sauce over the cod fillets.
6. Serve immediately.

Tips:

- For more savory meal, add a sprinkle of dried thyme or a dash of paprika before cooking.
- To make the meal extra creamy, add an additional tablespoon of olive oil before serving.
- For a richer meal, serve the cod fillets with a dollop of sour cream or Greek yogurt.

CRAB CURRY

- **Prep Time: 15 minutes**
- **Cooking Time: 20 minutes**
- **Serving Time: 5 minutes**
- **Total Time: 40 minutes**

NUTRITIONAL VALUE (PER SERVING):

- Calories: 300
- Fat: 15g
- Saturated Fat: 5g
- Carbohydrates: 15g
- Fiber: 4g
- Sugar: 10g
- Protein: 25g

INGREDIENTS:

- 1-pound lump crab meat
- 1 tablespoon olive oil
- 1 onion, chopped

- 2 cloves garlic, minced
- 1 tablespoon curry powder
- 1 (14-ounce) can coconut milk
- 1 cup vegetable broth
- 1/2 cup chopped fresh cilantro
- Salt and pepper to taste

INSTRUCTIONS:

1. Heat the olive oil in a large skillet or saucepan over medium heat.
2. Add the onion and simmer until softened, approximately 5 minutes.
3. Add the garlic and simmer for 1 minute longer.
4. Stir in the curry powder and simmer for 30 seconds, until aromatic.
5. Add the coconut milk, vegetable broth, crab meat, cilantro, salt, and pepper.
6. Bring to a boil, then decrease heat and simmer for 5-7 minutes, until the crab flesh is cooked through.
7. Serve immediately.

Tips:

- For a more delicious curry, add a touch of turmeric or a dash of ginger powder before cooking.
- To make the curry extra creamy, add an additional tablespoon of coconut milk before serving.
- For a healthy curry, use low-fat or dairy-free coconut milk.

SHRIMP WITH TOMATOES AND FETA

- **Prep Time: 10 minutes**
- **Cooking Time: 15 minutes**
- **Serving Time: 5 minutes**
- **Total Time: 30 minutes**

NUTRITIONAL VALUE (PER SERVING):

- Calories: 250
- Fat: 12g
- Saturated Fat: 4g
- Carbohydrates: 10g
- Fiber: 3g
- Sugar: 5g
- Protein: 25g

INGREDIENTS:

- 1-pound shrimp, peeled and deveined
- 1 tablespoon olive oil
- 1 onion, chopped
- 2 cloves garlic, minced
- 1 (14-ounce) can chopped tomatoes, undrained
- 1/2 cup crumbled feta cheese
- Salt and pepper to taste

INSTRUCTIONS:

1. Heat the olive oil in a large skillet or saucepan over medium heat.

2. Add the onion and simmer until softened, approximately 5 minutes.

3. Add the garlic and simmer for 1 minute longer.

4. Add the chopped tomatoes, feta cheese, shrimp, salt, and pepper.

5. Bring to a boil, then decrease heat and simmer for 5-7 minutes, or until the shrimp is cooked through.

6. Serve immediately.

SEAFOOD STEW

- **Prep Time: 15 minutes**
- **Cooking Time: 30 minutes**
- **Serving Time: 5 minutes**
- **Total Time: 50 minutes**

NUTRITIONAL VALUE (PER SERVING):

- Calories: 400
- Fat: 18g
- Saturated Fat: 6g
- Carbohydrates: 25g
- Fiber: 5g
- Sugar: 10g
- Protein: 35g

INGREDIENTS:

- 2 tablespoons olive oil
- 1 onion, chopped
- 2 cloves garlic, minced
- 1-pound cod fillets, cut into 1-inch pieces
- 1-pound shrimp, peeled and deveined
- 1 (14-ounce) can chopped tomatoes, undrained
- 1 (14-ounce) can vegetable broth
- 1 teaspoon dried thyme
- 1/2 teaspoon salt
- 1/4 teaspoon black pepper
- 1/4 cup chopped fresh parsley

INSTRUCTIONS:

1. Heat the olive oil in a big saucepan over medium heat.

2. Add the onion and simmer until softened, approximately 5 minutes.

3. Add the garlic and simmer for 1 minute longer.

4. Add the fish, shrimp, chopped tomatoes, vegetable broth, thyme, salt, and pepper.

5. Bring to a boil, then decrease heat and simmer for 20 minutes, or until the seafood is cooked through.

6. Stir in the parsley.

7. Serve immediately.

Tips:

- For more savory stew, add a touch of red pepper flakes or a dash of cayenne pepper before cooking.

- To make the stew extra creamy, add an additional tablespoon of olive oil before serving.
- For a thicker stew, add a dollop of sour cream or Greek yogurt to each dish.

SPICY CITRUS SOLE

- **Prep Time: 10 minutes**
- **Cooking Time: 15 minutes**
- **Serving Time: 5 minutes**
- **Total Time: 30 minutes**

NUTRITIONAL VALUE (PER SERVING):

- Calories: 250
- Fat: 10g
- Saturated Fat: 3g
- Carbohydrates: 5g
- Fiber: 1g
- Sugar: 3g
- Protein: 30g

INGREDIENTS:

- 2 lemon sole fillets
- 1 tablespoon olive oil
- 1/4 cup orange juice
- 1 tablespoon honey
- 1 teaspoon soy sauce
- 1 teaspoon chili powder
- 1/4 teaspoon salt
- 1/4 teaspoon black pepper

INSTRUCTIONS:

1. Preheat oven to 375 degrees F (190 degrees C).
2. Grease a 9x13-inch baking dish.
3. Pat the lemon sole fillets dry with paper towels.
4. In a small bowl, mix together the orange juice, honey, soy sauce, chili powder, salt, and pepper.
5. Place the lemon sole fillets in the prepared baking dish.
6. Pour the orange sauce over the lemon sole fillets.
7. Bake for 15 minutes, or until the lemon sole is cooked through.
8. Serve immediately.

Tips:

- For a more delicious meal, add a touch of ginger powder or a dash of garlic powder before cooking.
- To make the meal particularly hot, add an additional sprinkle of chili powder before cooking.
- For a richer meal, serve the lemon sole fillets with a dollop of sour cream or Greek yogurt.

HERB-CRUSTED HALIBUT

- **Prep Time: 15 minutes**
- **Cooking Time: 20 minutes**

Serving Time: 5 minutes

Total Time: 40 minutes

NUTRITIONAL VALUE (PER SERVING):

- Calories: 350
- Fat: 15g
- Saturated Fat: 5g
- Carbohydrates: 10g
- Fiber: 2g
- Sugar: 5g
- Protein: 35g

INGREDIENTS:

- 2 halibut fillets, approximately 6 ounces each
- 1 tablespoon olive oil
- 1/2 cup chopped fresh herbs (such as parsley, thyme, and oregano)
- 1/4 teaspoon salt
- 1/4 teaspoon black pepper

INSTRUCTIONS:

1. Preheat oven to 400 degrees F (200 degrees C).
2. In a small bowl, add the olive oil, herbs, salt, and pepper.
3. Place the halibut fillets on a baking sheet.
4. Spread the herb mixture evenly over the top of the halibut fillets.
5. Bake for 15-20 minutes, or until the halibut is cooked through.
6. Serve immediately.

Tips:

- For more savory crust, add a sprinkle of garlic powder or a dash of paprika to the herb mixture before spreading it over the halibut.
- To make the meal extra moist, baste the halibut fillets with olive oil or butter during baking.
- For a richer meal, serve the halibut fillets with a dollop of sour cream or Greek yogurt.

SALMON FLORENTINE

- **Prep Time: 10 minutes**
- **Cooking Time: 20 minutes**
- **Serving Time: 5 minutes**
- **Total Time: 35 minutes**

NUTRITIONAL VALUE (PER SERVING):

- Calories: 350
- Fat: 15g
- Saturated Fat: 5g
- Carbohydrates: 10g
- Fiber: 3g
- Sugar: 5g
- Protein: 35g

INGREDIENTS:

- 1-pound salmon fillets
- 1 tablespoon olive oil
- 1 (10-ounce) box frozen chopped spinach, thawed and drained
- 1/2 cup grated Parmesan cheese
- 1/4 cup chopped fresh basil
- 1 clove garlic, minced
- Salt and pepper to taste

INSTRUCTIONS:

1. Preheat oven to 400 degrees F (200 degrees C).
2. Grease a baking sheet with olive oil.
3. Place the salmon fillets on the prepared baking sheet.
4. In a medium bowl, mix the spinach, Parmesan cheese, basil, garlic, salt, and pepper.
5. Spread the spinach mixture evenly over the top of the salmon fillets.
6. Bake for 15-20 minutes, or until the salmon is cooked through and the spinach is heated through.
7. Serve immediately.

Tips:

- For more savory meal, add a sprinkle of dried oregano or a dash of red pepper flakes to the spinach mixture before spreading it over the salmon.
- To make the meal particularly creamy, add an additional tablespoon of olive oil to the spinach mixture before spreading it over the salmon.
- For a richer meal, serve the salmon with a dollop of sour cream or Greek yogurt.

SALMON CAKES IN AIR FRYER

- **Prep Time: 30 minutes**
- **Cooking Time: 10 minutes**
- **Serving Time: 5 minutes**
- **Total Time: 45 minutes**

NUTRITIONAL VALUE (PER SERVING):

- Calories: 250
- Fat: 12g
- Saturated Fat: 4g
- Carbohydrates: 5g
- Fiber: 2g
- Sugar: 4g
- Protein: 30g

INGREDIENTS:

- 1-pound salmon, cooked and flaked
- 1/2 cup panko bread crumbs
- 1/4 cup chopped fresh herbs (such as parsley, thyme, and oregano)
- 1/4 cup grated Parmesan cheese
- 1 egg
- 1 tablespoon olive oil
- Salt and pepper to taste

INSTRUCTIONS:

1. Preheat the air fryer to 375 degrees F (190 degrees C).

2. In a large bowl, mix the salmon, panko breadcrumbs, herbs, Parmesan cheese, egg, olive oil, salt, and pepper.

3. Mix until completely blended.

4. Form the salmon mixture into 4 patties.

5. Spray the air fryer basket with cooking spray.

6. Place the fish patties in the air fryer basket.

7. Cook for 10 minutes, or until golden brown and heated through.

8. Serve immediately.

Tips:

- For more savory dinner, add a touch of garlic powder or a dash of paprika to the salmon mixture before forming the patties.

- To make the patties extra moist, drizzle them with olive oil or butter while cooking.

- For a richer meal, serve the salmon patties with a dollop of sour cream or Greek yogurt.

COCONUT SHRIMP

- **Prep Time: 20 minutes**
- **Cooking Time: 10 minutes**
- **Serving Time: 5 minutes**
- **Total Time: 35 minutes**

NUTRITIONAL VALUE (PER SERVING):

- Calories: 300
- Fat: 18g
- Saturated Fat: 6g
- Carbohydrates: 15g
- Fiber: 5g
- Sugar: 10g
- Protein: 35g

INGREDIENTS:

- 1-pound shrimp, peeled and deveined
- 1 cup unsweetened coconut flakes
- 1/4 cup all-purpose flour
- 1/4 teaspoon salt
- 1/4 teaspoon black pepper

INSTRUCTIONS:

1. Preheat oven to 375 degrees F (190 degrees C).

2. Line a baking sheet with parchment paper.

3. In a medium bowl, mix the coconut flakes, flour, salt, and pepper.

4. Dredge the shrimp in the coconut mixture, covering evenly.

5. Place the shrimp on the prepared baking sheet.

6. Bake for 10-15 minutes, or until the shrimp is golden brown and cooked through.

7. Serve immediately with your favorite dipping sauce.

Tips:

- For a more delicious coating, add a sprinkle of curry powder or a dash of ginger powder to the coconut mixture before dredging the shrimp.
- To make the shrimp extra crispy, spray them with cooking spray before baking.
- For a richer meal, serve the coconut shrimp with a dollop of sour cream or Greek yogurt.

CRISPY FISH STICKS IN AIR FRYER

- **Prep Time: 15 minutes**
- **Cooking Time: 10 minutes**
- **Serving Time: 5 minutes**
- **Total Time: 30 minutes**

NUTRITIONAL VALUE (PER SERVING):

- Calories: 200
- Fat: 10g
- Saturated Fat: 3g
- Carbohydrates: 5g
- Fiber: 1g
- Sugar: 2g
- Protein: 25g

INGREDIENTS:

- 1-pound white fish fillets, cut into 1-inch strips
- 1/2 cup panko bread crumbs
- 1/4 cup grated Parmesan cheese
- 1 egg
- 1 tablespoon olive oil
- Salt and pepper to taste

INSTRUCTIONS:

1. Preheat the air fryer to 400 degrees F (200 degrees C).

2. In a large bowl, mix the panko breadcrumbs, Parmesan cheese, egg, olive oil, salt, and pepper.

3. Dredge the fish sticks in the breadcrumb mixture, covering evenly.

4. Spray the air fryer basket with cooking spray.

5. Place the fish sticks in the air fryer basket.

6. Cook for 8-10 minutes, or until golden brown and heated through.

7. Serve immediately with your favorite dipping sauce.

Tips:

- For a more delicious coating, add a sprinkle of garlic powder or a dash of paprika to the breadcrumb mixture before dredging the fish sticks.

- To make the fish sticks extra crispy, spray them with cooking spray before cooking.
- For a richer meal, serve the crispy fish sticks with a dollop of sour cream or Greek yogurt.

HONEY-GLAZED SALMON

- **Prep Time: 10 minutes**
- **Cooking Time: 15 minutes**
- **Serving Time: 5 minutes**
- **Total Time: 30 minutes**

NUTRITIONAL VALUE (PER SERVING):

- Calories: 300
- Fat: 15g
- Saturated Fat: 5g
- Carbohydrates: 5g
- Fiber: 1g
- Sugar: 5g
- Protein: 35g

INGREDIENTS:

- 1-pound salmon fillets
- 1/4 cup honey
- 2 teaspoons soy sauce
- 1 tablespoon Dijon mustard
- 1 clove garlic, minced
- Salt and pepper to taste

INSTRUCTIONS:

1. Preheat oven to 400 degrees F (200 degrees C).
2. Grease a baking sheet with olive oil.
3. In a small bowl, stir together the honey, soy sauce, Dijon mustard, garlic, salt, and pepper.
4. Place the salmon fillets on the prepared baking sheet.
5. Pour the honey glaze over the salmon fillets.
6. Bake for 12-15 minutes, or until the salmon is cooked through.
7. Serve immediately.

Tips:

- For a more delicious glaze, add a sprinkle of ginger powder or a dash of red pepper flakes to the honey glaze before pouring it over the salmon.
- To make the salmon moister, baste it with the honey glaze while baking.
- For a richer meal, serve the honey-glazed salmon with a dollop of sour cream or Greek yogurt.

BASIL-PARMESAN CRUSTED SALMON

- **Prep Time: 15 minutes**
- **Cooking Time: 15 minutes**
- **Serving Time: 5 minutes**
- **Total Time: 35 minutes**

NUTRITIONAL VALUE (PER SERVING):

- Calories: 350
- Fat: 18g
- Saturated Fat: 6g
- Carbohydrates: 5g
- Fiber: 1g
- Sugar: 3g
- Protein: 35g

INGREDIENTS:

- 1-pound salmon fillets
- 1/4 cup Parmesan cheese, grated
- 1/4 cup chopped fresh basil
- 1/4 teaspoon salt
- 1/4 teaspoon black pepper
- 1 tablespoon olive oil

INSTRUCTIONS:

1. Preheat oven to 400 degrees F (200 degrees C).
2. In a small bowl, add the Parmesan cheese, basil, salt, and pepper.
3. Place the salmon fillets on a baking sheet.
4. Spread the basil mixture equally over the top of each salmon fillet.
5. Drizzle with olive oil.
6. Bake for 12-15 minutes, or until the salmon is cooked through.
7. Serve immediately.

CAJUN SHRIMP IN AIR FRYER

- **Prep Time: 15 minutes**
- **Cooking Time: 10 minutes**
- **Serving Time: 5 minutes**
- **Total Time: 30 minutes**

NUTRITIONAL VALUE (PER SERVING):

- Calories: 300
- Fat: 20g
- Saturated Fat: 7g
- Carbohydrates: 10g
- Fiber: 2g
- Sugar: 5g
- Protein: 35g

INGREDIENTS:

- 1-pound shrimp, peeled and deveined
- 1/4 cup all-purpose flour
- 1 tablespoon Cajun seasoning
- 1/4 teaspoon salt
- 1/4 teaspoon black pepper
- 1 tablespoon olive oil

INSTRUCTIONS:

1. Preheat air fryer to 400 degrees F (200 degrees C).

2. In a medium bowl, mix the flour, Cajun spice, salt, and pepper.

3. Dredge the shrimp in the Cajun mixture, covering evenly.

4. Spray air fryer basket with cooking spray.

5. Place the shrimp in the air fryer basket.

6. Cook for 10 minutes, or until golden brown and heated through.

7. Serve immediately with your favorite dipping sauce.

Tips:

- For a savory supper, add a touch of paprika or a dash of dried oregano to the Cajun mixture before dredging the shrimp.
- To make the shrimp extra crispy, spray them with cooking spray before cooking.
- For a richer meal, serve the Cajun shrimp with a dollop of sour cream or Greek yogurt.
- Sure, here are the recipes for the remaining diabetic seafood dishes:

AIR-FRIED FISH NUGGETS

- **Prep Time: 15 minutes**
- **Cooking Time: 10 minutes**
- **Serving Time: 5 minutes**
- **Total Time: 30 minutes**

NUTRITIONAL VALUE (PER SERVING):

- Calories: 200
- Fat: 12g
- Saturated Fat: 4g
- Carbohydrates: 5g
- Fiber: 1g
- Sugar: 2g
- Protein: 25g

INGREDIENTS:

- 1-pound white fish fillets, cut into 1-inch pieces
- 1/2 cup panko bread crumbs
- 1/4 cup grated Parmesan cheese
- 1 egg
- 1 tablespoon olive oil
- Salt and pepper to taste

INSTRUCTIONS:

1. Preheat the air fryer to 400 degrees F (200 degrees C).

2. In a large bowl, mix the panko breadcrumbs, Parmesan cheese, egg, olive oil, salt, and pepper.

3. Dredge the fish nuggets in the breadcrumb mixture, covering evenly.

4. Spray the air fryer basket with cooking spray.

5. Place the fish nuggets in the air fryer basket.

6. Cook for 8-10 minutes, or until golden brown and heated through.

7. Serve immediately with your favorite dipping sauce.

Tips:

- For a more delicious coating, add a sprinkle of garlic powder or a dash of paprika to the breadcrumb mixture before dredging the fish nuggets.

- To make the fish nuggets extra crispy, spray them with cooking spray before cooking.

- For a richer meal, serve the air-fried fish nuggets with a dollop of sour cream or Greek yogurt.

GARLIC ROSEMARY GRILLED PRAWNS

- **Prep Time: 15 minutes**
- **Cooking Time: 5 minutes**
- **Serving Time: 5 minutes**
- **Total Time: 25 minutes**

NUTRITIONAL VALUE (PER SERVING):

- Calories: 250
- Fat: 10g
- Saturated Fat: 3g
- Carbohydrates: 5g
- Fiber: 1g
- Sugar: 2g
- Protein: 30g

INGREDIENTS:

- 1 pound prawns, peeled and deveined
- 2 tablespoons olive oil
- 2 cloves garlic, minced
- 1 teaspoon dried rosemary
- Salt and pepper to taste

INSTRUCTIONS:

1. Preheat grill or grill pan to medium-high heat.

2. In a large bowl, add the prawns, olive oil, garlic, rosemary, salt, and pepper.

3. Grill the prawns for 2-3 minutes each side, or until pink and cooked through.

4. Serve immediately with your favorite dipping sauce.

Tips:

- For a more delicious meal, marinate the prawns in the olive oil, garlic, rosemary, salt, and pepper combination for at least 30 minutes before grilling.

- To make the prawns juicier, baste them with the marinade while cooking.

- For a richer meal, serve the garlic rosemary grilled prawns with a dollop of sour cream or Greek yogurt.

AIR-FRIED CRUMBED FISH

- **Prep Time: 15 minutes**
- **Cooking Time: 10 minutes**
- **Serving Time: 5 minutes**
- **Total Time: 30 minutes**

NUTRITIONAL VALUE (PER SERVING):

- Calories: 250
- Fat: 12g
- Saturated Fat: 4g
- Carbohydrates: 10g
- Fiber: 2g
- Sugar: 2g
- Protein: 30g

INGREDIENTS:

- 1-pound white fish fillets
- 1/2 cup all-purpose flour
- 1/2 cup panko bread crumbs
- 1 teaspoon dried oregano
- 1/2 teaspoon salt
- 1/4 teaspoon black pepper
- 1 tablespoon olive oil

INSTRUCTIONS:

1. Preheat the air fryer to 400 degrees F (200 degrees C).
2. In a shallow bowl, mix the flour, panko breadcrumbs, oregano, salt, and pepper.
3. Dredge the salmon fillets in the flour mixture, covering evenly.
4. Spray the air fryer basket with cooking spray.
5. Place the fish fillets in the air fryer basket.
6. Cook for 8-10 minutes, or until golden brown and heated through.
7. Serve immediately with your favorite dipping sauce.

PARMESAN GARLIC CRUSTED SALMON

- **Prep Time: 15 minutes**
- **Cooking Time: 15 minutes**
- **Serving Time: 5 minutes**
- **Total Time: 35 minutes**

NUTRITIONAL VALUE (PER SERVING):

- Calories: 350
- Fat: 15g
- Saturated Fat: 5g
- Carbohydrates: 5g
- Fiber: 1g
- Sugar: 3g
- Protein: 35g

INGREDIENTS:

- 1-pound salmon fillets
- 1/4 cup Parmesan cheese, grated

- 1/4 cup chopped fresh parsley
- 1/4 teaspoon salt
- 1/4 teaspoon black pepper
- 1 tablespoon olive oil

INSTRUCTIONS:

1. Preheat oven to 400 degrees F (200 degrees C).
2. In a small bowl, add the Parmesan cheese, parsley, salt, and pepper.
3. Place the salmon fillets on a baking sheet.
4. Spread the parmesan mixture equally over the top of each salmon fillet.
5. Drizzle with olive oil.
6. Bake for 12-15 minutes, or until the salmon is cooked through.
7. Serve immediately.

Tips:

- For a more delicious crust, add a touch of garlic powder or a dash of red pepper flakes to the parmesan mixture before spreading it over the salmon.
- To make the crust extremely crispy, bake the salmon for an additional 2-3 minutes.
- For a richer meal, serve the parmesan garlic coated salmon with a dollop of sour cream or Greek yogurt.

AIR FRYER SALMON WITH MAPLE SOY GLAZE

- **Prep Time: 15 minutes**
- **Cooking Time: 10 minutes**
- **Serving Time: 5 minutes**
- **Total Time: 30 minutes**

NUTRITIONAL VALUE (PER SERVING):

- Calories: 300
- Fat: 12g
- Saturated Fat: 4g
- Carbohydrates: 10g
- Fiber: 2g
- Sugar: 4g
- Protein: 30g

INGREDIENTS:

- 1-pound salmon fillets
- 1/4 cup maple syrup
- 2 teaspoons soy sauce
- 1 tablespoon Dijon mustard
- 1 clove garlic, minced
- Salt and pepper to taste

INSTRUCTIONS:

1. Preheat air fryer to 400 degrees F (200 degrees C).
2. In a small bowl, mix together the maple syrup, soy sauce, Dijon mustard, garlic, salt, and pepper.

3. Place the salmon fillets in the air fryer basket.

4. Pour the maple soy glaze over the salmon fillets.

5. Cook for 10 minutes, or until the fish is cooked through.

6. Serve immediately.

Tips:

- For a more delicious glaze, add a sprinkle of ginger powder or a dash of red pepper flakes to the maple soy glaze before pouring it over the salmon.

- To make the salmon moister, baste it with the maple soy glaze while cooking.

- For a richer meal, serve the air fryer salmon with maple soy glaze with a dollop of sour cream or Greek yogurt.

AIR-FRIED CAJUN SALMON

- **Prep Time: 15 minutes**
- **Cooking Time: 10 minutes**
- **Serving Time: 5 minutes**
- **Total Time: 30 minutes**

NUTRITIONAL VALUE (PER SERVING):

- Calories: 350
- Fat: 18g
- Saturated Fat: 6g
- Carbohydrates: 5g
- Fiber: 1g
- Sugar: 3g
- Protein: 35g

INGREDIENTS:

- 1-pound salmon fillets
- 1/4 cup all-purpose flour
- 2 teaspoons Cajun seasoning
- 1/4 teaspoon salt
- 1/4 teaspoon black pepper
- 1 tablespoon olive oil

INSTRUCTIONS:

1. Preheat air fryer to 400 degrees F (200 degrees C).

2. In a small bowl, mix the flour, Cajun spice, salt, and pepper.

3. Dredge the salmon fillets in the flour mixture, covering evenly.

4. Spray the air fryer basket with cooking spray.

5. Place the salmon fillets in the air fryer basket.

6. Cook for 10 minutes, or until golden brown and heated through.

7. Serve immediately with your favorite dipping sauce.

Tips:

- For a more delicious coating, add a touch of paprika or a dash of dried oregano to the flour mixture before dredging the salmon fillets.

AIR FRYER SHRIMP SCAMPI

- **Prep Time: 15 minutes**
- **Cooking Time: 10 minutes**
- **Serving Time: 5 minutes**
- **Total Time: 30 minutes**

NUTRITIONAL VALUE (PER SERVING):

- Calories: 300
- Fat: 15g
- Saturated Fat: 5g
- Carbohydrates: 5g
- Fiber: 1g
- Sugar: 3g
- Protein: 30g

INGREDIENTS:

- 1-pound shrimp, peeled and deveined
- 2 tablespoons olive oil
- 3 cloves garlic, minced
- 1/4 cup dry white wine
- 1/4 cup chicken broth
- 1/4 cup chopped fresh parsley
- Salt and pepper to taste

INSTRUCTIONS:

1. Preheat air fryer to 400 degrees F (200 degrees C).
2. In a large bowl, add the shrimp, olive oil, garlic, white wine, chicken broth, parsley, salt, and pepper.
3. Toss to coat the shrimp evenly.
4. Place the shrimp in a single layer in the air fryer basket.
5. Cook for 10 minutes, or until the shrimp are pink and cooked through.
6. Serve immediately with your favorite dipping sauce.

Tips:

- For a savory meal, add a sprinkle of red pepper flakes to the shrimp mixture before cooking.
- To make the shrimp particularly juicy, baste them with the shrimp mixture while cooking.
- For a richer meal, serve the air fryer shrimp scampi with a dollop of sour cream or Greek yogurt.

SESAME SEED FISH FILLET

- **Prep Time: 10 minutes**
- **Cooking Time: 15 minutes**
- **Serving Time: 5 minutes**
- **Total Time: 30 minutes**

NUTRITIONAL VALUE (PER SERVING):

- Calories: 250
- Fat: 10g
- Saturated Fat: 3g
- Carbohydrates: 5g
- Fiber: 1g
- Sugar: 2g
- Protein: 30g

INGREDIENTS:

- 1-pound white fish fillets
- 1/4 cup soy sauce
- 1 tablespoon honey
- 1 tablespoon rice vinegar
- 1 tablespoon sesame oil
- 1 teaspoon minced ginger
- 1 clove garlic, minced
- 1/4 cup sesame seeds

INSTRUCTIONS:

1. In a shallow bowl, mix together the soy sauce, honey, rice vinegar, sesame oil, ginger, and garlic.
2. Place the fish fillets in the marinade, ensuring they are well covered.
3. Marinate for at least 15 minutes, or up to 2 hours.
4. Preheat oven to 400 degrees F (200 degrees C).
5. Spread the sesame seeds on a dish.
6. Dredge the salmon fillets in the sesame seeds, covering evenly.
7. Place the salmon fillets on a baking sheet lined with parchment paper.
8. Bake for 12-15 minutes, or until the fish is cooked through.
9. Serve immediately.

Tips:

- For a savory meal, add a touch of sriracha or a dash of red pepper flakes to the marinade before adding the fish fillets.
- To make the fish fillets extremely crispy, bake them for an additional 2-3 minutes.
- For a richer meal, serve the sesame seed fish fillet with a dollop of sour cream or Greek yogurt.

LEMON PEPPER SHRIMP IN THE AIR FRYER

- **Prep Time: 10 minutes**
- **Cooking Time: 10 minutes**
- **Serving Time: 5 minutes**
- **Total Time: 25 minutes**

NUTRITIONAL VALUE (PER SERVING):

- Calories: 250
- Fat: 12g
- Saturated Fat: 4g
- Carbohydrates: 5g

- Fiber: 1g
- Sugar: 2g
- Protein: 30g

INGREDIENTS:

- 1-pound shrimp, peeled and deveined
- 1 tablespoon olive oil
- 2 teaspoons lemon juice
- 1 tablespoon lemon zest
- 1 teaspoon black pepper
- 1/2 teaspoon salt

INSTRUCTIONS:

1. Preheat air fryer to 400 degrees F (200 degrees C).
2. In a large bowl, mix the shrimp, olive oil, lemon juice, lemon zest, black pepper, and salt.
3. Toss to coat the shrimp evenly.
4. Place the shrimp in a single layer in the air fryer basket.
5. Cook for 10-12 minutes, or until the shrimp are pink and cooked through.
6. Serve immediately with your favorite dipping sauce.

Tips:

- For a more delicious meal, add a touch of paprika or a dash of dried oregano to the shrimp combination before cooking.
- To make the shrimp particularly juicy, baste them with the shrimp mixture while cooking.
- For a richer meal, serve the lemon pepper shrimp in the air fryer with a dollop of sour cream or Greek yogurt.

MONKFISH CURRY

- **Prep Time: 20 minutes**
- **Cooking Time: 20 minutes**
- **Serving Time: 10 minutes**
- **Total Time: 50 minutes**

NUTRITIONAL VALUE (PER SERVING):

- Calories: 300
- Fat: 15g
- Saturated Fat: 5g
- Carbohydrates: 15g
- Fiber: 3g
- Sugar: 5g
- Protein: 30g

INGREDIENTS:

- 1-pound monkfish fillets, sliced into bite-sized portions
- 1 onion, finely chopped
- 2 cloves garlic, minced
- 1 tablespoon curry powder
- 1 teaspoon ground turmeric
- 1 teaspoon ground cumin

- 1/2 teaspoon ground ginger
- 1 (14-ounce) can chopped tomatoes
- 1 (14-ounce) can coconut milk
- Salt and pepper to taste
- Fresh cilantro for garnish (optional)

INSTRUCTIONS:

1. Heat the oil in a big saucepan over medium heat. Add the onion and simmer until softened, approximately 5 minutes.
2. Add the garlic, curry powder, turmeric, cumin, and ginger and sauté for 1 minute longer, until aromatic.
3. Stir in the chopped tomatoes and coconut milk. Bring to a simmer and cook for 10 minutes.
4. Add the monkfish and heat until cooked through, approximately 5 minutes.
5. Season with salt and pepper to taste.
6. Serve immediately over rice, topped with fresh cilantro if preferred.

Tips:

- For a more delicious curry, marinate the monkfish in the curry sauce for 30 minutes before cooking.
- To make the curry extremely hot, add a sprinkle of red pepper flakes to the curry sauce.
- For a richer meal, serve the monkfish curry with a dollop of sour cream or Greek yogurt.

SALMON BAKE

- **Prep Time: 15 minutes**
- **Cooking Time: 30 minutes**
- **Serving Time: 10 minutes**
- **Total Time: 55 minutes**

NUTRITIONAL VALUE (PER SERVING):

- Calories: 450
- Fat: 20g
- Saturated Fat: 6g
- Carbohydrates: 30g
- Fiber: 5g
- Sugar: 10g
- Protein: 40g

INGREDIENTS:

- 1-pound salmon fillets, skin on
- 1 tablespoon olive oil
- 1 onion, thinly sliced
- 2 carrots, finely sliced
- 2 celery stalks, thinly sliced
- 1 lemon, sliced
- 1/2 cup chicken broth
- 1/4 cup white wine
- 1 tablespoon dry herbs (such as thyme, oregano, and parsley)

Salt and pepper to taste

INSTRUCTIONS:

1. Preheat oven to 400 degrees F (200 degrees C).

2. Grease a baking dish with olive oil.

3. Place the salmon fillets in the prepared baking dish.

4. Arrange the onion, carrots, and celery around the fish.

5. Top with lemon slices.

6. In a small bowl, mix together the chicken broth, white wine, dried herbs, salt, and pepper.

7. Pour the broth mixture over the fish and veggies.

8. Bake for 30-35 minutes, or until the salmon is cooked through and the veggies are soft.

9. Serve immediately.

Tips:

- For a savory meal, add a touch of garlic powder or a dash of red pepper flakes to the broth combination.

- To make the veggies extra soft, pre-steam them for 5-10 minutes before putting them to the baking dish.

- For a richer meal, serve the salmon bake with a dollop of sour cream or Greek yogurt.

ROASTED SALMON WITH HONEY-MUSTARD SAUCE

- **Prep Time: 20 minutes**
- **Cooking Time: 15 minutes**
- **Serving Time: 10 minutes**
- **Total Time: 55 minutes**

NUTRITIONAL VALUE (PER SERVING):

- Calories: 400
- Fat: 20g
- Saturated Fat: 6g
- Carbohydrates: 25g
- Fiber: 5g
- Sugar: 10g
- Protein: 40g

INGREDIENTS:

- 1-pound salmon fillets, skin on
- 1 tablespoon olive oil
- 1/4 cup Dijon mustard
- 1 tablespoon honey
- 1 teaspoon lemon juice
- 1/2 teaspoon salt
- 1/4 teaspoon black pepper

INSTRUCTIONS:

1. Preheat oven to 400 degrees F (200 degrees C).

2. In a small bowl, mix together the olive oil, Dijon mustard, honey, lemon juice, salt, and pepper.

3. Place the salmon fillets on a baking sheet.

4. Brush the salmon fillets with the honey-mustard sauce.

5. Bake for 15-20 minutes, or until the salmon is cooked through and the sauce is slightly caramelized.

6. Serve immediately.

Tips:

- For a savory meal, add a sprinkle of garlic powder or a dash of red pepper flakes to the honey-mustard sauce.

- To make the salmon extra moist, coat the salmon fillets with the honey-mustard sauce again during the final 5 minutes of baking.

- For a richer meal, serve the roasted salmon with a dollop of sour cream or Greek yogurt.

ROASTED SALMON WITH SALSA VERDE

- **Prep Time: 20 minutes**
- **Cooking Time: 15 minutes**
- **Serving Time: 10 minutes**
- **Total Time: 55 minutes**

NUTRITIONAL VALUE (PER SERVING):

- Calories: 350
- Fat: 15g
- Saturated Fat: 5g
- Carbohydrates: 20g
- Fiber: 5g
- Sugar: 5g
- Protein: 40g

INGREDIENTS:

- 1-pound salmon fillets, skin on
- 1 cup salsa Verde
- Salt and pepper to taste

INSTRUCTIONS:

1. Preheat oven to 400 degrees F (200 degrees C).

2. In a small bowl, combine the salsa Verde with salt and pepper to taste.

3. Place the salmon fillets on a baking sheet.

4. Top each salmon fillet with a spoonful of the salsa Verde.

5. Bake for 15-20 minutes, or until the salmon is cooked through and the salsa Verde is gently heated through.

6. Serve immediately.

Tips:

- For a savory meal, add a sprinkle of cilantro or a dash of cumin to the salsa Verde.

- To make the salmon extra moist, baste the salmon fillets with the salsa Verde during the final 5 minutes of baking.

- For a richer meal, serve the roasted salmon with a dollop of sour cream or Greek yogurt.

SHRIMP WITH GREEN BEANS

- **Prep Time: 15 minutes**
- **Cooking Time: 10 minutes**
- **Serving Time: 5 minutes**
- **Total Time: 30 minutes**

NUTRITIONAL VALUE (PER SERVING):

- Calories: 250
- Fat: 12g
- Saturated Fat: 4g
- Carbohydrates: 5g
- Fiber: 2g
- Sugar: 2g
- Protein: 30g

INGREDIENTS:

- 1-pound shrimp, peeled and deveined
- 1 tablespoon olive oil
- 1 pound green beans, trimmed
- 1/2 cup sliced scallions
- 1 tablespoon soy sauce
- 1 tablespoon rice vinegar
- 1 teaspoon sesame oil
- Salt and pepper to taste

INSTRUCTIONS:

1. Preheat oven to 400 degrees F (200 degrees C).
2. In a large bowl, mix the shrimp with the olive oil, salt, and pepper.
3. Spread the shrimp on a baking sheet.
4. Bake for 5-7 minutes, or until the shrimp are pink and cooked through.
5. While the shrimp are baking, steam or blanch the green beans until tender-crisp.
6. In a large bowl, mix the cooked shrimp, steaming green beans, scallions, soy sauce, rice vinegar, and sesame oil.
7. Toss to coat evenly.
8. Serve immediately.

Tips:

- For a savory meal, add a touch of ginger powder or a dash of red pepper flakes to the shrimp and green bean combination.
- To make the meal more healthful, use brown rice vinegar instead of white rice vinegar.
- For a richer meal, serve the shrimp with a dollop of sour cream or Greek yogurt.

EGGPLANT PASTA

- **Prep Time: 15 minutes**
- **Cooking Time: 20 minutes**
- **Serving Time: 5 minutes**
- **Total Time: 40 minutes**

NUTRITIONAL VALUE (PER SERVING):

- Calories: 300
- Fat: 10g
- Saturated Fat: 3g
- Carbohydrates: 35g
- Fiber: 10g
- Sugar: 5g
- Protein: 15g

INGREDIENTS:

- 1 medium eggplant, cut into 1-inch cubes
- 1 tablespoon olive oil
- Salt and pepper to taste
- 1/2-pound whole-wheat pasta
- 1/4 cup chopped fresh parsley
- 1/4 cup grated Parmesan cheese

INSTRUCTIONS:

1. Preheat oven to 400 degrees F (200 degrees C).
2. Toss the eggplant cubes with the olive oil, salt, and pepper.
3. Spread the eggplant cubes on a baking sheet.
4. Bake for 20 minutes, or until the eggplant is soft and golden.
5. While the eggplant is baking, make the pasta according to package instructions.
6. Drain the pasta and toss it with the roasted eggplant, parsley, and Parmesan cheese.
7. Serve immediately.

Tip:

- For more savory meal, add a touch of garlic powder or a dash of red pepper flakes to the eggplant before roasting.
- To make the recipe extra healthful, use whole-wheat pasta instead of white spaghetti.
- For a richer meal, serve the eggplant spaghetti with a dollop of sour cream or Greek yogurt.

GARLIC PARMESAN ASPARAGUS

- **Prep Time: 10 minutes**
- **Cooking Time: 10 minutes**
- **Serving Time: 5 minutes**
- **Total Time: 25 minutes**

NUTRITIONAL VALUE (PER SERVING):

- Calories: 150
- Fat: 5g
- Saturated Fat: 2g
- Carbohydrates: 10g
- Fiber: 5g
- Sugar: 2g
- Protein: 5g

INGREDIENTS:

- 1-pound asparagus, trimmed
- 1 tablespoon olive oil
- 1/4 cup grated Parmesan cheese
- 1/4 teaspoon salt
- 1/4 teaspoon black pepper

INSTRUCTIONS:

1. Preheat oven to 400 degrees F (200 degrees C).
2. Toss the asparagus with the olive oil, Parmesan cheese, salt, and pepper.
3. Arrange the asparagus on a baking sheet.
4. Bake for 10 minutes, or until the asparagus is tender-crisp.
5. Serve immediately.

Tips:

- For more savory meal, add a touch of garlic powder or a dash of red pepper flakes to the asparagus before roasting.
- To make the meal particularly healthful, add Parmesan cheese sparingly.
- For a richer meal, serve the garlic Parmesan asparagus with a dollop of sour cream or Greek yogurt.

GREEN BEANS WITH SIZZLED GARLIC

- **Prep Time: 10 minutes**
- **Cooking Time: 10 minutes**
- **Serving Time: 5 minutes**
- **Total Time: 25 minutes**

NUTRITIONAL VALUE (PER SERVING):

- Calories: 100
- Fat: 5g
- Saturated Fat: 2g
- Carbohydrates: 10g
- Fiber: 5g
- Sugar: 2g
- Protein: 2g

INGREDIENTS:

- 1 pound green beans, trimmed
- 1 tablespoon olive oil
- 3 cloves garlic, minced
- Salt and pepper to taste

INSTRUCTIONS:

1. Heat the olive oil in a large pan over medium heat.

2. Add the garlic and simmer for 30 seconds, until fragrant.

3. Add the green beans and simmer for 5 minutes, or until tender-crisp.

4. Season with salt and pepper to taste.

5. Serve immediately.

Tips:

- For a more delicious meal, add a sprinkle of red pepper flakes to the garlic before cooking.

- To make the meal particularly nutritious, add olive oil sparingly.

- For a richer meal, serve the green beans with sizzled garlic with a dollop of sour cream or Greek yogurt.

GRILLED BROCCOLI STEAKS

- **Prep Time: 15 minutes**
- **Cooking Time: 15 minutes**
- **Serving Time: 5 minutes**
- **Total Time: 35 minutes**

NUTRITIONAL VALUE (PER SERVING):

- Calories: 120
- Fat: 5g
- Saturated Fat: 1g
- Carbohydrates: 10g
- Fiber: 5g
- Sugar: 3g
- Protein: 5g

INGREDIENTS:

- 2 big broccoli crowns, sliced into thick steaks
- 2 tablespoons olive oil
- 1 teaspoon salt
- 1/2 teaspoon black pepper

INSTRUCTIONS:

1. Preheat grill to medium-high heat.

2. Drizzle the broccoli steaks with olive oil and season with salt and pepper.

3. Grill the broccoli steaks for 10-15 minutes, or until tender-crisp and slightly browned.

4. Serve immediately.

Tips:

- For more savory dinner, coat the broccoli steaks with a balsamic glaze before grilling.

- To make the meal particularly nutritious, add olive oil sparingly.

- For a richer meal, serve the grilled broccoli steaks with a dollop of sour cream or Greek yogurt.

- **Prep Time: 15 minutes**
- **Cooking Time: 20 minutes**
- **Serving Time: 5 minutes**
- **Total Time: 40 minutes**

NUTRITIONAL VALUE (PER SERVING):

- Calories: 250
- Fat: 15g
- Saturated Fat: 5g
- Carbohydrates: 15g
- Fiber: 5g
- Sugar: 3g
- Protein: 10g

INGREDIENTS:

- 1 pound Brussels sprouts, trimmed and halved lengthwise
- 1 tablespoon olive oil
- Salt and pepper to taste
- 1/4 cup crumbled goat cheese
- 1/4 cup chopped walnuts

INSTRUCTIONS:

1. Preheat oven to 400 degrees F (200 degrees C).
2. Toss the Brussels sprouts with the olive oil, salt, and pepper.
3. Spread the Brussels sprouts on a baking sheet.
4. Roast for 20 minutes, or until the Brussels sprouts are soft and slightly browned.
5. Sprinkle with goat cheese and walnuts.
6. Serve immediately.

Tips:

- For more savory meal, add a touch of garlic powder or a dash of red pepper flakes to the Brussels sprouts before roasting.
- To make the meal particularly nutritious, add olive oil sparingly.
- For a richer meal, serve the roasted Brussels sprouts with goat cheese with a dollop of sour cream or Greek yogurt.

MUSHROOM & TOFU STIR FRY

- **Prep Time: 15 minutes**
- **Cooking Time: 10 minutes**
- **Serving Time: 5 minutes**
- **Total Time: 30 minutes**

NUTRITIONAL VALUE (PER SERVING):

- Calories: 250
- Fat: 10g
- Saturated Fat: 3g
- Carbohydrates: 20g
- Fiber: 5g

- Sugar: 3g
- Protein: 15g

INGREDIENTS:

- 1 pound mushrooms, sliced
- 1 block firm tofu, drained and cubed
- 1 tablespoon olive oil
- 1/4 cup low-sodium soy sauce
- 1 tablespoon rice vinegar
- 1 teaspoon sesame oil
- 1/4 teaspoon red pepper flakes (optional)

INSTRUCTIONS:

1. Heat the olive oil in a large pan or wok over medium-high heat.
2. Add the mushrooms and tofu and simmer for 5 minutes, or until the mushrooms are soft and the tofu is slightly browned.
3. Add the soy sauce, rice vinegar, sesame oil, and red pepper flakes (if using).
4. Cook for 2-3 minutes longer, until the sauce has thickened.
5. Serve immediately.

Tips:

- For more savory meal, add a touch of garlic powder or a dash of ginger powder to the tofu before cooking.
- To make the recipe extra nutritious, add low-sodium soy sauce.

- For a richer meal, serve the mushroom & tofu stir fry with a dollop of sour cream or Greek yogurt.

BAKED ZUCCHINI CHIPS

- **Prep Time: 15 minutes**
- **Cooking Time: 20 minutes**
- **Serving Time: 10 minutes**
- **Total Time: 45 minutes**

NUTRITIONAL VALUE (PER SERVING):

- Calories: 100
- Fat: 5g
- Saturated Fat: 1g
- Carbohydrates: 15g
- Fiber: 3g
- Sugar: 3g
- Protein: 2g

INGREDIENTS:

- 1 medium zucchini, finely sliced
- 1 tablespoon olive oil
- Salt and pepper to taste

INSTRUCTIONS:

1. Preheat oven to 200 degrees C (400 degrees F).
2. Line a baking sheet with parchment paper.

3. Arrange the zucchini slices on the prepared baking sheet.

4. Drizzle with olive oil and season with salt and pepper.

5. Bake for 20 minutes, or until the zucchini chips are golden brown and crispy.

6. Serve immediately.

Tips:

- For added flavor, add a sprinkle of garlic powder, paprika, or chili powder to the zucchini slices before baking.

- To make the zucchini chips extremely crispy, bake them for an additional 5-10 minutes.

- Serve the baked zucchini chips with your favorite dipping sauce, such as hummus, guacamole, or salsa.

BLACK BEAN TORTILLA WRAPS

- **Prep Time: 10 minutes**
- **Cooking Time: 10 minutes**
- **Serving Time: 5 minutes**
- **Total Time: 25 minutes**

NUTRITIONAL VALUE (PER SERVING):

- Calories: 300
- Fat: 10g
- Saturated Fat: 3g
- Carbohydrates: 40g
- Fiber: 10g
- Sugar: 5g
- Protein: 10g

INGREDIENTS:

- 1 (15-ounce) can black beans, drained and rinsed
- 1/4 cup chopped onion
- 1/4 cup chopped red bell pepper
- 1 tablespoon olive oil
- 1 teaspoon chili powder
- 1/2 teaspoon cumin
- 1/4 teaspoon salt
- 1/4 teaspoon black pepper
- 4 whole-wheat tortillas

INSTRUCTIONS:

1. In a medium bowl, mash the black beans using a fork.

2. Add the onion, red bell pepper, olive oil, chili powder, cumin, salt, and pepper.

3. Mix thoroughly to mix.

4. Spread the black bean mixture equally across the tortillas.

5. Roll up the tortillas and serve immediately.

Tips:

- For added flavor, add a sprinkle of garlic powder or oregano to the black bean mixture.

- To make the wraps more filling, add shredded cheese, lettuce, or sliced tomatoes.

- Serve the black bean tortilla wraps with a side of salsa, sour cream, or guacamole.

ASPARAGUS-TOFU STIR FRY

- **Prep Time: 15 minutes**
- **Cooking Time: 10 minutes**
- **Serving Time: 5 minutes**
- **Total Time: 30 minutes**

NUTRITIONAL VALUE (PER SERVING):

- Calories: 250
- Fat: 10g
- Saturated Fat: 3g
- Carbohydrates: 20g
- Fiber: 5g
- Sugar: 5g
- Protein: 15g

INGREDIENTS:

- 1-pound asparagus, trimmed
- 1 block firm tofu, drained and cubed
- 1 tablespoon olive oil
- 1/4 cup low-sodium soy sauce
- 1 tablespoon rice vinegar
- 1 teaspoon sesame oil
- 1/4 teaspoon red pepper flakes (optional)

INSTRUCTIONS:

1. Heat the olive oil in a large pan or wok over medium-high heat.
2. Add the asparagus and tofu and simmer for 5 minutes, or until the asparagus is tender-crisp and the tofu is slightly browned.
3. Add the soy sauce, rice vinegar, sesame oil, and red pepper flakes (if using).
4. Cook for 2-3 minutes longer, until the sauce has thickened.
5. Serve immediately.

Tips:

- For added flavor, add a sprinkle of garlic powder or ginger powder to the tofu before cooking.

- To make the recipe extra nutritious, add low-sodium soy sauce.

- Serve the asparagus-tofu stir fry with a dollop of sour cream or Greek yogurt, if preferred.

BLACK BEAN-ORANGE CHILI

- **Prep Time: 15 minutes**

- **Cooking Time: 30 minutes**
- **Serving Time: 10 minutes**
- **Total Time: 55 minutes**

NUTRITIONAL VALUE (PER SERVING):

- Calories: 350
- Fat: 15g
- Saturated Fat: 5g
- Carbohydrates: 35g
- Fiber: 10g
- Sugar: 5g
- Protein: 15g

INGREDIENTS:

- 1 (15-ounce) can black beans, drained and rinsed
- 1 (14.5-ounce) can chopped tomatoes
- 1 (15-ounce) can tomato sauce
- 1 cup vegetable broth
- 1/4 cup chopped onion
- 1/4 cup chopped green bell pepper
- 2 cloves garlic, minced
- 1 tablespoon chili powder
- 1 teaspoon cumin
- 1/2 teaspoon oregano
- 1/4 teaspoon salt
- 1/4 teaspoon black pepper
- 1 orange, zested and juiced
- 1 tablespoon honey
- Cilantro leaves, for garnish (optional)

INSTRUCTIONS:

1. In a large saucepan, add the black beans, chopped tomatoes, tomato sauce, vegetable broth, onion, green bell pepper, garlic, chili powder, cumin, oregano, salt, and pepper.
2. Bring to a boil, then decrease heat and simmer for 20 minutes, or until the chili has thickened.
3. Stir in the orange zest, orange juice, and honey.
4. Simmer for 5 minutes longer, or until the flavors have merged.
5. Serve immediately, garnished with cilantro leaves if preferred.

Tips:

- For added flavor, add a sprinkle of cayenne pepper or smoky paprika to the chili.
- To make the chili spicier, add a couple diced jalapeño peppers.
- Serve the black bean-orange chili with a dollop of sour cream or Greek yogurt, if preferred.

CUMIN QUINOA PATTIES

- **Prep Time: 15 minutes**
- **Cooking Time: 20 minutes**
- **Serving Time: 5 minutes**
- **Total Time: 40 minutes**

- Calories: 300
- Fat: 10g
- Saturated Fat: 3g
- Carbohydrates: 35g
- Fiber: 10g
- Sugar: 5g
- Protein: 15g

INGREDIENTS:

- 1 cup cooked quinoa
- 1/4 cup chopped onion
- 1/4 cup chopped red bell pepper
- 1/4 cup chopped cilantro
- 1/4 cup chopped walnuts
- 1 tablespoon olive oil
- 1 tablespoon lemon juice
- 1 teaspoon cumin
- 1/2 teaspoon salt
- 1/4 teaspoon black pepper

INSTRUCTIONS:

1. In a large bowl, mix the quinoa, onion, red bell pepper, cilantro, walnuts, olive oil, lemon juice, cumin, salt, and pepper.
2. Mash the contents together with a fork until fully incorporated.
3. Form the mixture into 4-6 patties.
4. Heat a large skillet over medium heat.
5. Add the patties to the skillet and cook for 5 minutes each side, or until golden brown and crispy.
6. Serve immediately.

Tips:

- For added flavor, add a sprinkle of garlic powder or chile powder to the patties.
- To make the patties extra crispy, pan-fry them for an additional 1-2 minutes each side.
- Serve the cumin quinoa patties with your favorite dip, such as salsa, guacamole, or hummus.

KALE QUESADILLAS

- **Prep Time: 10 minutes**
- **Cooking Time: 10 minutes**
- **Serving Time: 5 minutes**
- **Total Time: 25 minutes**

NUTRITIONAL VALUE (PER SERVING):

- Calories: 300
- Fat: 15g
- Saturated Fat: 5g
- Carbohydrates: 30g
- Fiber: 10g
- Sugar: 5g
- Protein: 10g

INGREDIENTS:

- 2 whole-wheat tortillas
- 1 cup chopped kale
- 1/4 cup chopped red onion
- 1/4 cup shredded cheese
- 1 tablespoon olive oil

INSTRUCTIONS:

1. Spread one side of each tortilla with olive oil.
2. Arrange the kale, red onion, and cheese on one side of each tortilla.
3. Fold the tortillas in half.
4. Heat a large skillet over medium heat.
5. Place the quesadillas in the pan and cook for 3-4 minutes each side, or until golden brown and the cheese has melted.
6. Cut the quesadillas into wedges and serve immediately.

Tips:

- For added flavor, add a sprinkle of garlic powder, paprika, or chili powder to the kale combination.
- To make the quesadillas extra full, add chopped tomatoes, avocado, or cooked beans to the kale mixture.
- Serve the kale quesadillas with a dollop of sour cream or Greek yogurt, if preferred.

QUINOA-STUFFED ZUCCHINI

- **Prep Time: 20 minutes**
- **Cooking Time: 30 minutes**
- **Serving Time: 10 minutes**
- **Total Time: 60 minutes**

NUTRITIONAL VALUE (PER SERVING):

- Calories: 400
- Fat: 15g
- Saturated Fat: 5g
- Carbohydrates: 45g
- Fiber: 15g
- Sugar: 5g
- Protein: 15g

INGREDIENTS:

2 medium zucchini, split lengthwise and hollowed out

1 cup cooked quinoa

1/2 cup chopped onion

1/2 cup chopped red bell pepper

- 1/4 cup chopped tomatoes
- 1/4 cup chopped fresh parsley
- 1 tablespoon olive oil
- 1 teaspoon lemon juice
- 1/2 teaspoon salt
- 1/4 teaspoon black pepper

INSTRUCTIONS:

1. Preheat oven to 350 degrees F (175 degrees C).

2. In a large bowl, add the quinoa, onion, red bell pepper, tomatoes, parsley, olive oil, lemon juice, salt, and pepper.

3. Stuff the quinoa mixture into the hollowed-out zucchini halves.

4. Place the packed zucchini in a baking dish.

5. Bake for 30 minute, or until the zucchini is soft and the quinoa is cooked through.

Tips:

- For added flavor, add a sprinkle of garlic powder, cumin, or oregano to the quinoa mixture.

- To make the recipe extra cheesy, add grated cheese to the quinoa mixture before filling the zucchini.

- Serve the quinoa-stuffed zucchini with a side salad or steamed veggies.

QUINOA WITH VEGETABLE STIR FRY

- **Prep Time: 15 minutes**
- **Cooking Time: 20 minutes**
- **Serving Time: 5 minutes**
- **Total Time: 40 minutes**

NUTRITIONAL VALUE (PER SERVING):

- Calories: 350
- Fat: 15g
- Saturated Fat: 5g
- Carbohydrates: 40g
- Fiber: 10g
- Sugar: 5g
- Protein: 15g

INGREDIENTS:

- 1 cup cooked quinoa
- 1 tablespoon olive oil
- 1 cup chopped broccoli florets
- 1 cup sliced carrots
- 1/2 cup chopped red bell pepper
- 1/4 cup chopped onion
- 1 tablespoon soy sauce
- 1 tablespoon rice vinegar
- 1 teaspoon sesame oil
- Salt and pepper to taste

INSTRUCTIONS:

1. Heat the olive oil in a large pan or wok over medium-high heat.

2. Add the broccoli, carrots, red bell pepper, and onion.

3. Cook for 5 minutes, or until the veggies are tender-crisp.

4. Add the quinoa, soy sauce, rice vinegar, sesame oil, salt, and pepper.

5. Stir to incorporate and simmer for 2-3 minutes longer, until the sauce is cooked through.

6. Serve immediately.

- For added flavor, add a sprinkle of garlic powder or ginger powder to the veggies before cooking.

- To make the meal particularly spicy, add a sprinkle of red pepper flakes to the sauce.

- Serve the quinoa with veggie stir fry with a dollop of sour cream or Greek yogurt, if preferred.

Reciepe Card

COURSE:

DIET:

PREP TIME:

COOK TIME:

SERVINGS

INSTRUCTIONS

INGREDIENTS

Serves

Prep

Cook Time

TIPS & TRICKS

NOTES

ALMOND COCONUT BISCOTTI

- **Prep Time: 15 minutes**
- **Cooking Time: 20 minutes**
- **Serving Time: 5 minutes**
- **Total Time: 40 minutes**

NUTRITIONAL VALUE:

- Calories: 150
- Fat: 10g
- Saturated Fat: 3g
- Carbohydrates: 10g
- Fiber: 2g
- Sugar: 3g
- Protein: 3g

INGREDIENTS:

- 1 cup almond flour
- 1/2 cup shredded coconut
- 1/4 cup granulated sugar replacement
- 1/4 cup almond milk
- 1 egg
- 1 teaspoon vanilla extract
- 1/4 teaspoon salt

INSTRUCTIONS:

1. Preheat oven to 350 degrees F (175 degrees C).
2. In a large bowl, mix together the almond flour, coconut, sugar replacement, almond milk, egg, vanilla extract, and salt.
3. Drop by rounded spoonful onto ungreased baking sheets.
4. Bake for 10 minutes, or until softly golden brown.
5. Remove from oven and allow cool for 5 minutes.
6. Cut each biscuit into 3 biscotti.
7. Place biscotti back on baking pans and bake for an additional 5 minutes, or until golden brown and crisp.
8. Let cool fully before storing.

Tips:

- For added flavor, add a pinch of almond extract or cinnamon to the dough.
- To make the biscotti extra crispy, bake them for an additional 2-3 minutes each side.
- Store biscotti in an airtight jar at room temperature.

CHEESY TACO BITES

- **Prep Time: 10 minutes**
- **Cooking Time: 15 minutes**
- **Serving Time: 5 minutes**
- **Total Time: 30 minutes**

NUTRITIONAL VALUE:

- Calories: 100

- Fat: 5g
- Saturated Fat: 2g
- Carbohydrates: 5g
- Fiber: 1g
- Sugar: 1g
- Protein: 3g

INGREDIENTS:

- 1 cup shredded cheddar cheese
- 1/4 cup ground beef
- 1/4 cup chopped onion
- 1/4 cup chopped green bell pepper
- 1 tablespoon taco seasoning
- 1/4 cup low-carb tortillas, cut into 12 circles

INSTRUCTIONS:

1. Preheat oven to 350 degrees F (175 degrees C).
2. In a large bowl, add the cheese, ground beef, onion, green bell pepper, and taco spice.
3. Spoon 1 spoonful of the mixture onto each tortilla circle.
4. Place tortillas on a baking sheet.
5. Bake for 15 minutes, or until the cheese is melted and bubbling.
6. Serve immediately.

Tips:

- For added flavor, add a sprinkle of chili powder or cumin to the meat mixture.
- To make the bits extremely spicy, add a sprinkle of red pepper flakes to the beef mixture.
- Serve the cheesy taco bits with a dab of sour cream or Greek yogurt, if preferred.

ALMOND FLOUR CRACKERS

- **Prep Time: 10 minutes**
- **Cooking Time: 15 minutes**
- **Serving Time: 5 minutes**
- **Total Time: 30 minutes**

NUTRITIONAL VALUE:

- Calories: 50
- Fat: 3g
- Saturated Fat: 1g
- Carbohydrates: 2g
- Fiber: 1g
- Sugar: 1g
- Protein: 2g

INGREDIENTS:

- 1 cup almond flour
- 1/4 teaspoon salt
- 2 tablespoons olive oil
- 2 tablespoons water

INSTRUCTIONS:

1. Preheat oven to 350 degrees F (175 degrees C).

2. In a large basin, mix together the almond flour and salt.

3. Stir in the olive oil and water until a dough forms.

4. Roll the dough out on a lightly floured board to 1/8-inch thickness.

5. Cut the dough into squares or preferred shapes.

6. Place the crackers on a baking sheet.

7. Bake for 15 minutes, or until softly golden brown.

8. Let cool fully before storing.

CRACKERS

- **Prep Time: 10 minutes**
- **Cooking Time: 10 minutes**
- **Serving Time: 5 minutes**
- **Total Time: 25 minutes**

NUTRITIONAL VALUE:

- Calories: 55
- Fat: 4g
- Saturated Fat: 1g
- Carbohydrates: 1g
- Fiber: 1g
- Sugar: 1g
- Protein: 1g

INGREDIENTS:

- 1/2 cup almond flour
- 1/4 cup unsweetened shredded coconut
- 1/4 teaspoon salt
- 2 tablespoons butter, melted
- 1 tablespoon unsweetened almond milk

INSTRUCTIONS:

1. Preheat oven to 350 degrees F (175 degrees C).

2. In a large basin, mix together the almond flour, coconut, and salt.

3. Stir in the melted butter and almond milk until a dough forms.

4. Roll the dough out on a lightly floured board to 1/8-inch thickness.

5. Cut the dough into squares or preferred shapes.

6. Place the crackers on a baking sheet.

7. Bake for 10 minutes, or until softly golden brown.

8. Let cool fully before storing.

Tips:

- For added flavor, add a sprinkle of cinnamon or chocolate powder to the dough.
- To make the crackers extremely crispy, bake them for an additional 2-3 minutes each side.

ASIAN CHICKEN WINGS

- **Prep Time: 20 minutes**
- **Cooking Time: 30 minutes**
- **Serving Time: 5 minutes**
- **Total Time: 55 minutes**

NUTRITIONAL VALUE:

- Calories: 250
- Fat: 15g
- Saturated Fat: 5g
- Carbohydrates: 2g
- Fiber: 1g
- Sugar: 0g
- Protein: 20g

INGREDIENTS:

- 1-pound chicken wings
- 1/4 cup soy sauce
- 1/4 cup honey
- 1 tablespoon rice vinegar
- 1 tablespoon sesame oil
- 1 tablespoon grated ginger
- 1 tablespoon minced garlic
- 1/4 teaspoon red pepper flakes

INSTRUCTIONS:

1. Preheat oven to 400 degrees F (200 degrees C).
2. In a large bowl, add the soy sauce, honey, rice vinegar, sesame oil, ginger, garlic, and red pepper flakes.
3. Add the chicken wings to the marinade and toss to coat.
4. Place the chicken wings on a baking sheet.
5. Bake for 30 minutes, or until the chicken is cooked through and the sauce has thickened.
6. Serve immediately.

Tips:

- For added flavor, add a sprinkle of sesame seeds or scallions to the chicken wings before serving.
- To make the chicken wings extra crispy, broil them for an additional 5-10 minutes each side.

BANANA NUT COOKIES

- **Prep Time: 10 minutes**
- **Cooking Time: 12 minutes**
- **Serving Time: 5 minutes**
- **Total Time: 27 minutes**

NUTRITIONAL VALUE:

- Calories: 90
- Fat: 4g
- Saturated Fat: 2g
- Carbohydrates: 13g
- Fiber: 2g
- Sugar: 10g
- Protein: 2g

INGREDIENTS:

- 1 cup mashed ripe banana
- 1/2 cup almond flour
- 1/4 cup chopped walnuts
- 1 tablespoon honey
- 1 teaspoon vanilla extract
- 1/4 teaspoon salt

INSTRUCTIONS:

1. Preheat oven to 350 degrees F (175 degrees C).
2. In a large basin, mash the banana.
3. Stir in the almond flour, walnuts, honey, vanilla essence, and salt until a dough forms.
4. Drop by rounded spoonful onto ungreased baking sheets.
5. Bake for 12 minutes, or until golden brown.
6. Let cool fully before storing.

Tips:

- For added flavor, add a sprinkle of cinnamon or chocolate chips to the dough.
- To make the cookies chewier, bake them

BLT STUFFED CUCUMBERS

- **Prep Time: 10 minutes**
- **Cooking Time: 10 minutes**
- **Serving Time: 5 minutes**
- **Total Time: 25 minutes**

NUTRITIONAL VALUE:

- Calories: 80
- Fat: 5g
- Saturated Fat: 2g
- Carbohydrates: 5g
- Fiber: 2g
- Sugar: 1g
- Protein: 3g

INGREDIENTS:

- 1 cucumber, halved lengthwise and hollowed out
- 2 slices cooked bacon, diced
- 1/4 cup chopped lettuce
- 1/4 cup chopped tomato
- 1 tablespoon mayonnaise
- Salt and pepper to taste

INSTRUCTIONS:

1. Fill the cucumber halves with the lettuce, tomato, bacon, and mayonnaise.
2. Season with salt and pepper to taste.
3. Serve immediately.

Tips:

- For added flavor, add a sprinkle of onion powder or garlic powder to the filling.

- To make the filled cucumbers more full, add a piece of cheese to each half.

BUFFALO BITES

- **Prep Time: 15 minutes**
- **Cooking Time: 20 minutes**
- **Serving Time: 10 minutes**
- **Total Time: 45 minutes**

NUTRITIONAL VALUE:

- Calories: 200
- Fat: 12g
- Saturated Fat: 4g
- Carbohydrates: 5g
- Fiber: 1g
- Sugar: 2g
- Protein: 10g

INGREDIENTS:

- 1 pound boneless, skinless chicken breasts, cooked and chopped
- 1/2 cup spicy sauce
- 1/4 cup low-fat blue cheese crumbles
- 1/4 cup chopped celery
- 1 tablespoon mayonnaise
- Salt and pepper to taste

INSTRUCTIONS:

1. In a large bowl, mix the chicken, spicy sauce, blue cheese crumbles, celery, and mayonnaise.
2. Season with salt and pepper to taste.
3. Form the mixture into 12 balls.
4. Place the balls on a baking sheet lined with parchment paper.
5. Bake for 20 minutes, or until the buffalo bits are cooked through.
6. Serve immediately.

Tips:

- For added taste, add a sprinkle of garlic powder or onion powder to the filling.
- To make the buffalo bits spicier, add a sprinkle of cayenne pepper to the hot sauce.
- Serve the buffalo bits with a side of celery sticks or carrot sticks.

SALTED MACADAMIA KETO BOMBS

- **Prep Time: 5 minutes**
- **Cooking Time: 10 minutes**
- **Serving Time: 5 minutes**
- **Total Time: 20 minutes**

NUTRITIONAL VALUE:

- Calories: 200
- Fat: 18g
- Saturated Fat: 3g
- Carbohydrates: 3g
- Fiber: 1g

- Sugar: 1g
- Protein: 3g

INGREDIENTS:

- 1/2 cup unsweetened macadamia nuts
- 1/4 cup unsweetened shredded coconut
- 1/4 cup unsweetened cocoa powder
- 1/4 cup powdered erythritol
- 1/4 teaspoon salt

INSTRUCTIONS:

1. In a food processor, blend the macadamia nuts, coconut, cocoa powder, and erythritol.
2. Pulse until the mixture is finely ground.
3. Add the salt and pulse until mixed.
4. Roll the mixture into 12 balls.
5. Place the balls on a baking sheet lined with parchment paper.
6. Freeze for 10 minutes, or until the balls are firm.
7. Serve immediately.

Tips:

- For added flavor, add a pinch of vanilla extract or cinnamon to the mixture.
- To make the keto bombs really chocolaty, add a few drops of unsweetened chocolate stevia to the recipe.

- Dip the keto bombs in melted dark chocolate for an added delight.

PISTACHIO AND COCOA SQUARES

- **Prep Time: 15 minutes**
- **Cooking Time: 10 minutes**
- **Serving Time: 5 minutes**
- **Total Time: 30 minutes**

NUTRITIONAL VALUE (PER SERVING):

- Calories: 200
- Fat: 12g
- Saturated Fat: 2g
- Carbohydrates: 10g
- Fiber: 2g
- Sugar: 4g
- Protein: 4g

INGREDIENTS:

- 1/2 cup unsalted pistachios, chopped
- 1/4 cup unsweetened cocoa powder
- 1/4 cup almond flour
- 1/4 cup powdered erythritol
- 1/4 teaspoon salt
- 1/4 cup unsweetened almond milk

INSTRUCTIONS:

1. Preheat oven to 350°F (175°C). Line an 8x8 baking dish with parchment paper.

2. In a food processor, blend the pistachios, chocolate powder, almond flour, erythritol, and salt. Pulse until the mixture is finely ground.

3. Add the almond milk and pulse until a dough forms.

4. Press the dough evenly into the prepared baking dish.

5. Bake for 10-12 minutes, or until the edges are firm and the centers are slightly soft.

6. Let cool fully before cutting into squares.

Tips:

- For added taste, add a sprinkle of cinnamon or nutmeg to the mixture.
- To make the squares extra chewy, bake for an additional 2-3 minutes.
- Store the squares in an airtight jar in the refrigerator for up to 2 weeks.

PEPPERMINT AND CHOCOLATE KETO SQUARES

- **Prep Time: 10 minutes**
- **Cooking Time: 10 minutes**
- **Serving Time: 5 minutes**
- **Total Time: 25 minutes**

NUTRITIONAL VALUE (PER SERVING):

- Calories: 250
- Fat: 18g
- Saturated Fat: 4g
- Carbohydrates: 4g
- Fiber: 1g
- Sugar: 1g
- Protein: 3g

INGREDIENTS:

- 1/2 cup unsweetened shredded coconut
- 1/4 cup unsweetened cocoa powder
- 1/4 cup powdered erythritol
- 1/4 teaspoon peppermint extract
- 1/4 teaspoon salt
- 2 tablespoons unsweetened dark chocolate chips, melted

INSTRUCTIONS:

1. Line an 8x8 baking dish with parchment paper.

2. In a medium dish, mix the coconut, cocoa powder, erythritol, peppermint extract, and salt.

3. Press the mixture evenly into the prepared baking dish.

4. Drizzle the melted chocolate chips over the top of the mixture.

5. Refrigerate for at least 30 minutes, or until the chocolate has firm.

6. Cut into squares and enjoy!

- For added flavor, add a sprinkle of cinnamon or almond essence to the mixture.
- To make the squares really chocolaty, add one additional tablespoon of melted chocolate chips.
- Dip the squares in melted dark chocolate for an added delight.

GINGER PATTIES

- **Prep Time: 10 minutes**
- **Cooking Time: 15 minutes**
- **Serving Time: 5 minutes**
- **Total Time: 30 minutes**

NUTRITIONAL VALUE (PER SERVING):

- Calories: 150
- Fat: 8g
- Saturated Fat: 2g
- Carbohydrates: 10g
- Fiber: 2g
- Sugar: 4g
- Protein: 2g

INGREDIENTS:

- 1 cup unsweetened shredded coconut
- 1/4 cup almond flour
- 1/4 cup powdered erythritol
- 1 teaspoon ground ginger
- 1/4 teaspoon salt
- 1 tablespoon unsweetened almond milk

INSTRUCTIONS:

1. Preheat oven to 350°F (175°C). Line a baking sheet with parchment paper.
2. In a medium bowl, mix the coconut, almond flour, erythritol, ginger, and salt.
3. Add the almond milk and stir until a dough forms.
4. Drop rounded portions of the dough onto the prepared baking sheet.
5. Bake for 15-17 minutes, or until the sides are golden brown and the centers are firm.
6. Let cool fully before storing

Reciepe Card

COURSE: DIET: PREP TIME: COOK TIME: SERVINGS

INSTRUCTIONS

INGREDIENTS

Serves   Prep   Cook Time

TIPS & TRICKS

NOTES

COCOA MOUSSE

- **Prep Time: 10 minutes**
- **Serving Time: 5 minutes**
- **Cooking Time: None**

NUTRITIONAL VALUES PER SERVING:

- Calories: 160
- Fat: 10 grams
- Saturated Fat: 5 grams
- Carbohydrates: 15 grams
- Fiber: 2 grams
- Sugar: 10 grams
- Protein: 4 grams

INGREDIENTS:

- 1/2 cup thick cream
- 1/4 cup unsweetened cocoa powder
- 1/4 cup powdered erythritol
- 1/4 teaspoon vanilla extract
- Pinch of salt

INSTRUCTIONS:

1. In a large bowl, beat the heavy cream until firm peaks form.
2. In a separate dish, mix together the cocoa powder, powdered erythritol, vanilla extract, and salt.
3. Gently whisk the chocolate mixture into the whipped cream until just incorporated.
4. Divide the mousse among serving glasses or bowls.
5. Refrigerate for at least 30 minutes before serving.

Tips:

- For a deeper taste, use dark chocolate cocoa powder.
- To make the mousse more delicious, top with a dollop of whipped cream and a sprinkling of chocolate powder.
- Store the remaining mousse in an airtight jar in the refrigerator for up to 3 days.

COCONUT ICE CREAM

- **Prep Time: 10 minutes**
- **Serving Time: 5 minutes**
- **Cooking Time: 2 hours**

NUTRITIONAL VALUES PER SERVING:

- Calories: 200
- Fat: 14 grams
- Saturated Fat: 10 grams
- Carbohydrates: 18 grams
- Fiber: 2 grams
- Sugar: 12 grams
- Protein: 2 grams

INGREDIENTS:

- 1 can (14 ounces) full-fat coconut milk
- 1/4 cup powdered erythritol
- 1/4 teaspoon vanilla extract
- Pinch of salt

INSTRUCTIONS:

1. In a large bowl, mix together the coconut milk, powdered erythritol, vanilla extract, and salt.
2. Pour the ingredients into an ice cream maker and churn according to the manufacturer's directions.
3. Transfer the ice cream to an airtight container and freeze for at least 2 hours before serving.

Tips:

- For a creamier texture, add a spoonful of unsweetened almond milk to the mixture before churning.
- To make the ice cream tastier, add a sprinkle of cinnamon or nutmeg to the mixture before churning.
- Store the remaining ice cream in an airtight jar in the freezer for up to 1 month.

CHOCO-NUT MILKSHAKE

- **Prep Time: 5 minutes**
- **Serving Time: 5 minutes**
- **Cooking Time: None**

NUTRITIONAL VALUES PER SERVING:

- Calories: 280
- Fat: 16 grams
- Saturated Fat: 8 grams
- Carbohydrates: 25 grams
- Fiber: 3 grams
- Sugar: 18 grams
- Protein: 10 grams

INGREDIENTS:

- 1 cup unsweetened almond milk
- 1/4 cup unsweetened shredded coconut
- 1/4 cup unsweetened cocoa powder
- 1/4 cup powdered erythritol
- 1 teaspoon vanilla extract
- Pinch of salt

INSTRUCTIONS:

- In a blender, mix the almond milk, shredded coconut, cocoa powder, powdered erythritol, vanilla extract, and salt.
- Blend until smooth and creamy.
- Serve immediately.

Tips:

- For a thicker milkshake, add a couple more ice cubes to the blender.

- To make the milkshake particularly chocolatey, add a couple teaspoons of unsweetened dark chocolate chips to the blender.
- Store the remaining milkshake in an airtight jar in the refrigerator for up to 2 days.

RASPBERRY & MANGO SMOOTHIE

- **Prep Time: 5 minutes**
- **Serving Time: 5 minutes**
- **Cooking Time: None**

NUTRITIONAL VALUES PER SERVING:

- Calories: 190
- Fat: 12 grams
- Saturated Fat: 5 grams
- Carbohydrates: 22 grams
- Fiber: 4 grams
- Sugar: 16 grams
- Protein: 7 grams

INGREDIENTS:

- 1 cup frozen raspberries
- 1 cup frozen mango chunks
- 1/2 cup unsweetened almond milk
- 1/4 cup powdered erythritol
- 1 teaspoon vanilla extract
- Pinch of salt

INSTRUCTIONS:

- In a blender, add the frozen raspberries, frozen mango chunks, almond milk, powdered erythritol, vanilla extract, and salt.
- Blend until smooth and creamy.
- Serve immediately.

Tips:

- For a sweeter smoothie, add a couple more teaspoons of powdered erythritol.
- To make the smoothie more refreshing, add a few ice cubes to the blender.
- Store the remaining smoothie in an airtight jar in the refrigerator for up to 2 days.

CANTALOUPE SMOOTHIE

- **Prep Time: 5 minutes**
- **Serving Time: 5 minutes**
- **Cooking Time: None**

NUTRITIONAL VALUES PER SERVING:

- Calories: 180
- Fat: 11 grams
- Saturated Fat: 6 grams
- Carbohydrates: 21 grams
- Fiber: 3 grams

- Sugar: 15 grams
- Protein: 6 grams

INGREDIENTS:

- 1 cup frozen cantaloupe chunks
- 1/2 cup unsweetened almond milk
- 1/4 cup powdered erythritol
- 1 teaspoon vanilla extract
- Pinch of salt

INSTRUCTIONS:

1. In a blender, mix the frozen cantaloupe pieces, almond milk, powdered erythritol, vanilla extract, and salt.
2. Blend until smooth and creamy.
3. Serve immediately.

Tips:

- For a sweeter smoothie, add a couple more teaspoons of powdered erythritol.
- To make the smoothie more refreshing, add a few ice cubes to the blender.
- Store the remaining smoothie in an airtight jar in the refrigerator for up to 2 days.

BERRY & SPINACH SMOOTHIE

- **Prep Time: 5 minutes**
- **Serving Time: 5 minutes**
- **Cooking Time: None**

NUTRITIONAL VALUES PER SERVING:

- Calories: 210
- Fat: 13 grams
- Saturated Fat: 7 grams
- Carbohydrates: 25 grams
- Fiber: 4 grams
- Sugar: 19 grams
- Protein: 8 grams

INGREDIENTS:

- 1 cup frozen mixed berries
- 1 cup spinach
- 1/2 cup unsweetened almond milk
- 1/4 cup powdered erythritol
- 1 teaspoon vanilla extract

INSTRUCTIONS:

1. In a blender, combine the frozen mixed berries, spinach, almond milk, powdered erythritol, and vanilla extract.
2. Blend until smooth and creamy.
3. Serve immediately.

Tips:

- For a sweeter smoothie, add a couple more teaspoons of powdered erythritol.

- To make the smoothie more refreshing, add a few ice cubes to the blender.
- Store the remaining smoothie in an airtight jar in the refrigerator for up to 2 days.

BRULEE ORANGES

- **Prep Time: 15 minutes**
- **Serving Time: 5 minutes**
- **Cooking Time: 20 minutes**

NUTRITIONAL VALUES PER SERVING:

- Calories: 160
- Fat: 4 grams
- Saturated Fat: 2 grams
- Carbohydrates: 32 grams
- Fiber: 3 grams
- Sugar: 28 grams
- Protein: 1 gram

INGREDIENTS:

- 2 oranges
- ¼ cup granulated erythritol
- 2 teaspoons unsweetened almond milk
- 1 teaspoon vanilla extract
- Pinch of salt

INSTRUCTIONS:

1. Preheat oven to 350 degrees F (175 degrees C).
2. Cut the oranges in half horizontally and scoop out the meat, leaving behind the rind.
3. In a small bowl, mix together the granulated erythritol, almond milk, vanilla extract, and salt.
4. Pour the mixture into the orange halves and bake for 15-20 minutes, or until the erythritol has melted and slightly caramelized.
5. Let cool fully before serving.

Tips:

- For a more robust taste, add a sprinkle of cinnamon or nutmeg to the mixture.
- To make the brulee oranges particularly spectacular, top with a dollop of whipped cream and a sprig of fresh mint.
- Store the remaining brulee oranges in an airtight jar in the refrigerator for up to 2 days.

FROZEN BLUEBERRY LEMONADE

- **Prep Time: 10 minutes**
- **Serving Time: 5 minutes**
- **Cooking Time: None**

- Calories: 120
- Fat: 1 gram
- Saturated Fat: 0 grams
- Carbohydrates: 29 grams
- Fiber: 2 grams
- Sugar: 27 grams
- Protein: 1 gram

INGREDIENTS:

- 1 cup frozen blueberries
- ½ cup unsweetened lemon juice
- ¼ cup powdered erythritol
- 1 cup unsweetened sparkling water

INSTRUCTIONS:

1. In a blender, mix the frozen blueberries, lemon juice, and powdered erythritol.
2. Blend until smooth and creamy.
3. Add the sparkling water and whisk until mixed.
4. Serve immediately.

Tips:

- For a sweeter lemonade, add a couple more teaspoons of powdered erythritol.
- To make the lemonade more refreshing, pour it over ice.

- Store the remaining lemonade in an airtight jar in the freezer for up to 2 days.

PEANUT BUTTER CHOCO CHIP COOKIES

- **Prep Time: 15 minutes**
- **Serving Time: 5 minutes**
- **Cooking Time: 10-12 minutes**

NUTRITIONAL VALUES PER SERVING (2 COOKIES):

- Calories: 220
- Fat: 14 grams
- Saturated Fat: 7 grams
- Carbohydrates: 23 grams
- Fiber: 2 grams
- Sugar: 16 grams
- Protein: 4 grams

INGREDIENTS:

- 1 cup unsweetened almond flour
- ¼ cup powdered erythritol
- ¼ teaspoon salt
- ½ cup unsweetened natural peanut butter
- 1 teaspoon vanilla extract
- ¼ cup unsweetened dark chocolate chips, melted

INSTRUCTIONS:

1. Preheat oven to 350 degrees F (175 degrees C). Line a baking sheet with parchment paper.
2. In a medium bowl, mix together the almond flour, powdered erythritol, and salt.
3. In a separate dish, mix together the peanut butter and vanilla extract.
4. Add the wet ingredients to the dry components and stir until a dough forms.
5. Stir in the chocolate chips.
6. Drop rounded portions of the dough onto the prepared baking sheet.
7. Bake for 10-12 minutes, or until the edges are golden brown.
8. Let cool fully before storing.

WATERMELON SHERBET

- **Prep Time: 10 minutes**
- **Serving Time: 5 minutes**
- **Cooking Time: None**

NUTRITIONAL VALUES PER SERVING (1/2 CUP):

- Calories: 120
- Fat: 2 grams
- Saturated Fat: 1 gram
- Carbohydrates: 28 grams
- Fiber: 2 grams
- Sugar: 26 grams
- Protein: 1 gram

INGREDIENTS:

- 2 cups seedless watermelon, frozen
- ¼ cup powdered erythritol
- Pinch of salt

INSTRUCTIONS:

1. In a blender, mix the frozen watermelon, powdered erythritol, and salt.
2. Blend until smooth and creamy.
3. Serve immediately.

Tips:

- For a sweeter sherbet, add a couple more teaspoons of powdered erythritol.
- To make the sherbet more refreshing, add a couple ice cubes to the blender.
- Store the remaining sherbet in an airtight jar in the freezer for up to 2 weeks.

NO-BAKE CHOCOLATE CHEESECAKE

- **Prep Time: 15 minutes**
- **Serving Time: 5 minutes**
- **Cooking Time: None**

NUTRITIONAL VALUES PER SERVING:

- Calories: 250
- Fat: 18 grams
- Saturated Fat: 10 grams
- Carbohydrates: 23 grams
- Fiber: 3 grams
- Sugar: 16 grams
- Protein: 7 grams

INGREDIENTS:

- 1 ½ cups almond flour
- ¼ cup unsweetened cocoa powder
- ¼ cup powdered erythritol
- ¼ teaspoon salt
- ½ cup unsweetened almond butter
- 2 teaspoons unsweetened almond milk
- 1 teaspoon vanilla extract
- 1 tablespoon unsweetened chopped dark chocolate

INSTRUCTIONS:

1. In a medium bowl, mix together the almond flour, cocoa powder, powdered erythritol, and salt.
2. In a separate dish, mix together the almond butter, almond milk, and vanilla extract.
3. Add the wet ingredients to the dry components and stir until a dough forms.
4. Press the dough into an 8-inch pie plate.
5. Melt the dark chocolate and drizzle over the top.
6. Refrigerate for at least 2 hours before serving.

Tips:

- For a deeper taste, use dark chocolate cocoa powder.
- To make the cheesecake more delicious, top with a dollop of whipped cream and a dusting of chocolate powder.
- Store the remaining cheesecake in an airtight jar in the refrigerator for up to 5 days.

EASY KETO CHOCOLATE MOUSSE

- **Prep Time: 10 minutes**
- **Serving Time: 5 minutes**
- **Cooking Time: None**

NUTRITIONAL VALUES PER SERVING:

- Calories: 180
- Fat: 14 grams
- Saturated Fat: 8 grams
- Carbohydrates: 4 grams
- Fiber: 2 grams
- Sugar: 3 grams
- Protein: 6 grams

INGREDIENTS:

- ¾ cup thick cream
- 2 teaspoons unsweetened cocoa powder
- 2 teaspoons powdered erythritol
- ¼ teaspoon vanilla extract
- Pinch of salt

INSTRUCTIONS:

1. In a large bowl, beat the heavy cream until firm peaks form.
2. In a separate dish, mix together the cocoa powder, powdered erythritol, vanilla extract, and salt.
3. Gently whisk the chocolate mixture into the whipped cream until just incorporated.
4. Divide the mousse among serving glasses or bowls.
5. Refrigerate for at least 30 minutes before serving.

Tips:

- For a deeper taste, use dark chocolate cocoa powder.
- To make the mousse more delicious, top with a dollop of whipped cream and a sprinkling of chocolate powder.
- Store the remaining mousse in an airtight jar in the refrigerator for up to 2 days.

KETO STRAWBERRY SHORTCAKE

- **Prep Time: 15 minutes**
- **Serving Time: 5 minutes**
- **Cooking Time: 10-12 minutes**

NUTRITIONAL VALUES PER SERVING:

- Calories: 240
- Fat: 18 grams
- Saturated Fat: 12 grams
- Carbohydrates: 17 grams
- Fiber: 3 grams
- Sugar: 10 grams
- Protein: 6 grams

INGREDIENTS:

- 1 cup almond flour
- ¼ cup powdered erythritol
- ¼ teaspoon salt
- ½ cup unsweetened almond butter
- 1 teaspoon vanilla extract
- 1 cup fresh strawberries, sliced
- ¼ cup unsweetened whipped cream

INSTRUCTIONS:

1. Preheat oven to 350 degrees F (175 degrees C). Line a baking sheet with parchment paper.
2. In a medium bowl, mix together the almond flour, powdered erythritol, and salt.

3. In a separate dish, mix together the almond butter and vanilla extract.

4. Add the wet ingredients to the dry components and stir until a dough forms.

5. Divide the dough into 6 equal pieces and make into biscuits.

6. Place the biscuits on the prepared baking sheet and bake for 10-12 minutes, or until golden brown.

7. Let cool fully before assembly.

8. To assemble, top each biscuit with a dollop of whipped cream and a layer of strawberries.

KETO CHOCOLATE DONUTS

- **Prep Time: 20 minutes**
- **Serving Time: 5 minutes**
- **Cooking Time: 8-10 minutes**

NUTRITIONAL VALUES PER SERVING:

- Calories: 220
- Fat: 15 grams
- Saturated Fat: 8 grams
- Carbohydrates: 18 grams
- Fiber: 3 grams
- Sugar: 10 grams
- Protein: 7 grams

INGREDIENTS:

- 1 cup almond flour
- ¼ cup unsweetened cocoa powder
- ¼ cup powdered erythritol
- ¼ teaspoon baking soda
- Pinch of salt
- 2 big eggs
- ¼ cup unsweetened almond milk
- 2 tablespoons unsweetened melted chocolate, for coating

INSTRUCTIONS:

1. Preheat oven to 350 degrees F (175 degrees C). Grease a donut pan with frying spray.

2. In a medium bowl, mix together the almond flour, cocoa powder, powdered erythritol, baking soda, and salt.

3. In a separate dish, mix together the eggs and almond milk.

4. Pour the wet ingredients into the dry ingredients and stir until barely mixed.

5. Spoon the batter into the prepared donut pan, filling each donut hole approximately ¾ full.

6. Bake for 8-10 minutes, or until a toothpick inserted into the middle comes out clean.

7. Let cool in the donut pan for a few minutes before transferring to a wire rack to cool fully.

8. Dip the cooled donuts in the melted chocolate, letting the excess drop off.

KETO RASPBERRY CHEESECAKE BARS

- **Prep Time: 20 minutes**
- **Serving Time: 5 minutes**
- **Cooking Time: 30-35 minutes**

NUTRITIONAL VALUES PER SERVING (1 BAR):

- Calories: 250
- Fat: 17 grams
- Saturated Fat: 10 grams
- Carbohydrates: 16 grams
- Fiber: 4 grams
- Sugar: 9 grams
- Protein: 8 grams

INGREDIENTS:

- 1 ½ cups almond flour
- ½ cup powdered erythritol
- ¼ teaspoon salt
- ½ cup unsweetened almond butter
- 1 big egg
- 1 teaspoon vanilla extract
- 1 cup fresh raspberries
- ¼ cup unsweetened heavy cream

INSTRUCTIONS:

1. Preheat oven to 350 degrees F (175 degrees C). Line an 8x8 inch baking tray with parchment paper.
2. In a medium bowl, mix together the almond flour, powdered erythritol, and salt.
3. Add the almond butter, egg, and vanilla essence and stir until a dough forms.
4. Press the dough into the prepared baking pan.
5. Bake for 10-12 minutes, or until the crust is golden brown.
6. Let cool fully while making the topping.
7. In a blender, add the raspberries and heavy cream and blend until smooth.
8. Spread the raspberry mixture over the chilled crust.
9. Refrigerate for at least 2 hours before slicing and serving.

KETO TIRAMISU

- **Prep Time: 15 minutes**
- **Serving Time: 5 minutes**
- **Cooking Time: None**

NUTRITIONAL VALUES PER SERVING:

- Calories: 280
- Fat: 17 grams

- Saturated Fat: 10 grams
- Carbohydrates: 12 grams
- Fiber: 2 grams
- Sugar: 6 grams
- Protein: 12 grams

INGREDIENTS:

- 1 cup unsweetened heavy cream
- ½ cup unsweetened cocoa powder
- ¼ cup powdered erythritol
- ¼ teaspoon vanilla extract
- Pinch of salt
- 12 ladyfingers
- ½ cup unsweetened brewed espresso
- 2 tablespoons unsweetened chocolate chips, melted

INSTRUCTIONS:

1. In a large bowl, beat the heavy cream until firm peaks form.
2. In a separate dish, mix together the cocoa powder, powdered erythritol, vanilla extract, and salt.
3. Gently whisk the chocolate mixture into the whipped cream until just incorporated.
4. Dip each ladyfinger in the espresso and then place them in a single layer in a 9x13 inch baking dish.
5. Spread half of the cocoa mixture over the ladyfingers.
6. Repeat the dipping and layering procedure with the remaining ladyfingers and cocoa mixture.
7. Drizzle the melted chocolate chips over the top.
8. Refrigerate for at least 2 hours before serving.

KETO CHOCOLATE AVOCADO MOUSSE

- **Prep Time: 10 minutes**
- **Serving Time: 5 minutes**
- **Cooking Time: None**

NUTRITIONAL VALUES PER SERVING:

- Calories: 200
- Fat: 16 grams
- Saturated Fat: 7 grams
- Carbohydrates: 7 grams
- Fiber: 6 grams
- Sugar: 3 grams
- Protein: 5 grams

INGREDIENTS:

- 1 ripe avocado
- ¼ cup unsweetened cocoa powder
- ¼ cup powdered erythritol
- ¼ teaspoon vanilla extract
- Pinch of salt
- 2 teaspoons unsweetened heavy cream

INSTRUCTIONS:

1. In a blender or food processor, mix the avocado, chocolate powder, powdered erythritol, vanilla extract, and salt.

2. Blend until smooth and creamy.

3. Slowly add the heavy cream while continuing to mix until a mousse-like consistency is obtained.

4. Divide the mousse among serving glasses or bowls.

5. Refrigerate for at least 30 minutes before serving.

KETO LEMON BARS

- **Prep Time: 20 minutes**
- **Serving Time: 5 minutes**
- **Cooking Time: 30-35 minutes**

NUTRITIONAL VALUES PER SERVING:

- Calories: 220
- Fat: 14 grams
- Saturated Fat: 8 grams
- Carbohydrates: 15 grams
- Fiber: 3 grams
- Sugar: 9 grams
- Protein: 6 grams

INGREDIENTS:

- 1 ½ cups almond flour
- ½ cup powdered erythritol
- ¼ teaspoon salt
- ½ cup unsweetened almond butter
- 1 big egg
- 1 teaspoon vanilla extract
- ¼ cup unsweetened lemon juice
- 1 tablespoon unsweetened heavy cream

INSTRUCTIONS:

1. Preheat oven to 350 degrees F (175 degrees C). Line a 9x13 inch baking pan with parchment paper.

2. In a medium bowl, mix together the almond flour, powdered erythritol, and salt.

3. Add the almond butter, egg, and vanilla essence and stir until a dough forms.

4. Press the dough into the prepared baking pan.

5. Bake for 10-12 minutes, or until the crust is golden brown.

6. Let cool fully while making the topping.

7. In a small bowl, mix together the lemon juice and heavy cream.

8. Pour the lemon mixture over the cooled crust and bake for an additional 15-20 minutes, or until the topping is set.

9. Refrigerate for at least 2 hours before slicing and serving.

Understanding Diabetes:

1. **What is diabetes?**

   A. Diabetes is a chronic condition where your body either doesn't produce enough insulin or doesn't use it effectively, leading to high blood sugar levels.

2. **What are the different types of diabetes?**

   A. There are three main types: Type 1 (autoimmune), Type 2 (lifestyle-related), and Gestational (pregnancy-related).

3. **What are the symptoms of diabetes?**

   A. Common symptoms include excessive thirst, frequent urination, fatigue, blurry vision, slow-healing wounds, and unexplained weight loss.

4. **How is diabetes diagnosed?**

   A. Blood tests like A1C, fasting blood sugar, and oral glucose tolerance test are used to diagnose diabetes.

Managing Diabetes:

5. **What is the treatment for diabetes?**

   A. Treatment varies but often includes a combination of healthy diet, regular exercise, blood sugar monitoring, and medication (if needed).

6. **Can I eat sugar if I have diabetes?**

   A. You can still enjoy occasional treats, but focus on a balanced diet rich in fruits, vegetables, whole grains, and lean protein. Read labels carefully and limit refined sugars.

7. **Can I exercise with diabetes?**

   A. Regular physical activity is crucial for managing blood sugar and overall health. Choose activities you enjoy and start slowly, consulting your doctor if needed.

8. **How often should I check my blood sugar?**

   A. Your doctor will advise on the recommended frequency based on your type and severity of diabetes.

9. **What are the long-term complications of diabetes?**

   A. Uncontrolled diabetes can lead to heart disease, stroke, kidney problems, nerve damage, and vision loss.

10. **Can I prevent diabetes?**

    A. While not guaranteed, maintaining a healthy weight, eating balanced meals, exercising regularly, and managing stress can significantly reduce your risk of developing diabetes.

11. **Is there a cure for diabetes?**

    A. Currently, there is no cure, but effective management can prevent complications and greatly improve quality of life.

Lifestyle and Support:

12. **Can I travel with diabetes?**

    A. Yes, but plan ahead. Pack your medications, blood sugar monitoring supplies, and healthy snacks. Inform airlines and travel insurance about your needs.

13. **How can I manage diabetes during pregnancy?**

    A. Consult your doctor for specialized care and maintain healthy habits. Gestational diabetes usually resolves after childbirth, but monitor for future risk.

14. **How can I cope with emotional challenges of diabetes?**

    A. Living with diabetes can be stressful. Seek support from family, friends, or a diabetes support group. Consider therapy to manage emotional well-being.

15. **What resources are available for people with diabetes?**

    A. Numerous organizations and online resources offer information, support groups, and other resources to help you manage your diabetes effectively.

Technology and Monitoring:

16. **What are continuous glucose monitoring (CGM) systems?**

    A. CGMs provide real-time blood sugar readings through a sensor inserted under the skin. This can help you make informed decisions about food, exercise, and medication.

17. **Are there apps available to help manage diabetes?**

    A. Many apps can track blood sugar levels, log meals and exercise, set reminders for medication, and offer educational resources.

18. **What are the latest advancements in diabetes technology?**

   A. Research is ongoing in areas like artificial pancreas systems, closed-loop insulin delivery systems, and even stem cell therapy.

19. **Are there foods I should completely avoid?**

   A. Focus on balanced meals and moderate portion sizes. While limiting sugary drinks and processed foods is crucial, most foods can be enjoyed in moderation with planning.

20. **What are some healthy substitutions for sugary ingredients?**

   A. Use natural sweeteners like stevia, erythritol, or monk fruit extract instead of sugar. Choose unsweetened yogurt, applesauce, or mashed banana for baking.

21. **Are there diabetic-friendly recipes available?**

   A. Numerous cookbooks and online resources offer delicious and nutritious recipes specifically designed for diabetic meal plans.

22. **Can I still eat out with diabetes?**

   A. Yes, ask restaurants about nutritional information and choose healthier options like grilled fish, chicken, salads, and whole grains.

23. **Can diabetes affect my mental health?**

   A. Living with diabetes can lead to anxiety, depression, and fear of complications. Talk to your doctor about available mental health support services.

24. **How can I find a diabetes support group?**

   A. Check with your local hospital, diabetes organizations, or online communities to connect with others who understand your struggles.

25. **How can I stay motivated to manage my diabetes?**

   A. Set realistic goals, celebrate small victories, and reward yourself for progress. Find partners for exercise or meal planning to stay accountable.

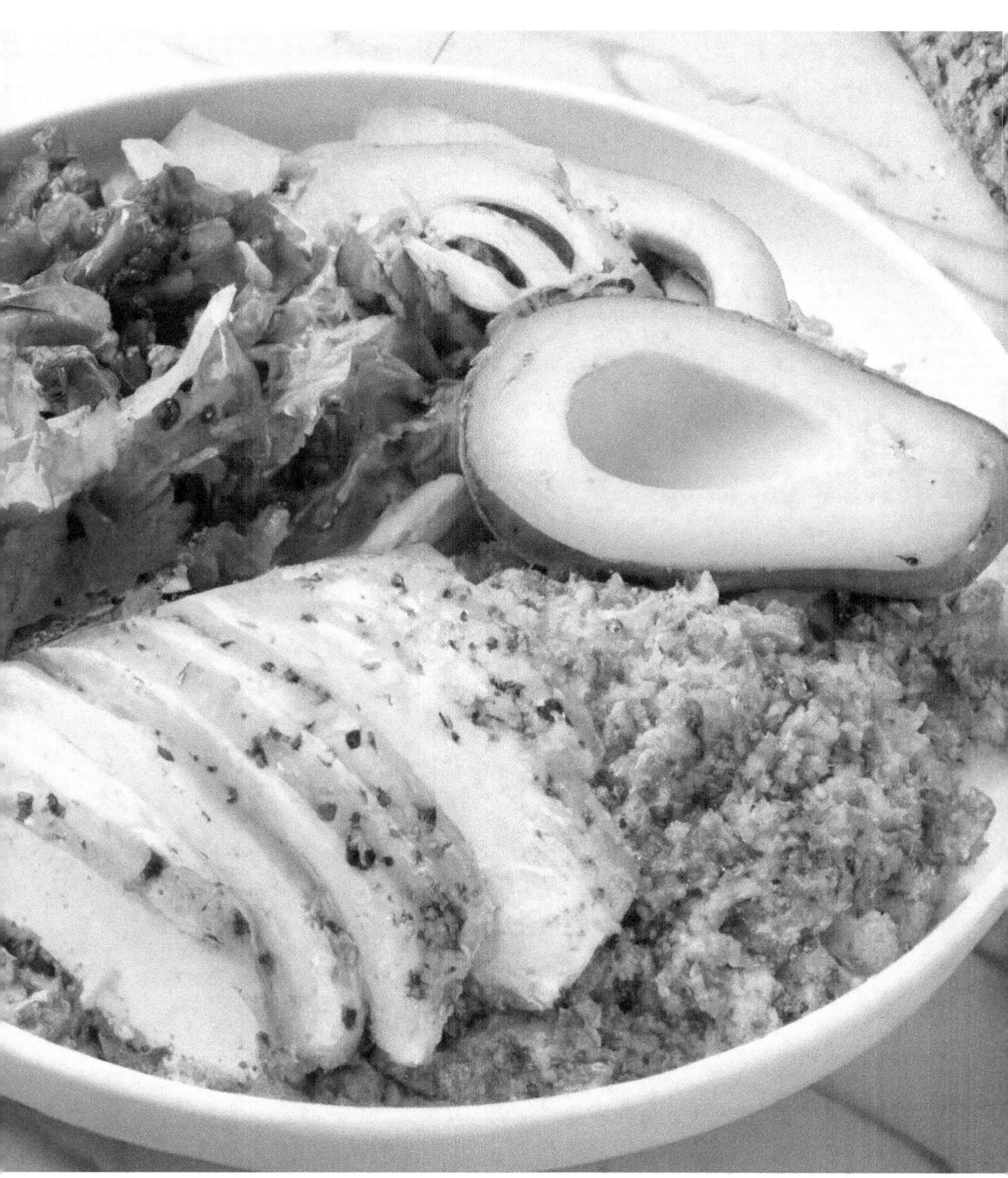